SpringerBriefs in Electrical and Computer Engineering

More information about this series at http://www.springer.com/series/10059

Fabian Gigengack • Xiaoyi Jiang
Mohammad Dawood • Klaus P. Schäfers

Motion Correction in Thoracic Positron Emission Tomography

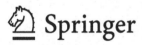
Springer

Fabian Gigengack
Department of Mathematics
and Computer Science
University of Münster
Münster, Germany

Mohammad Dawood
European Institute for Molecular
Imaging
University of Münster
Münster, Germany

Xiaoyi Jiang
Department of Mathematics
and Computer Science
University of Münster
Münster, Germany

Klaus P. Schäfers
European Institute for Molecular
Imaging
University of Münster
Münster, Germany

ISSN 2191-8112   ISSN 2191-8120 (electronic)
ISBN 978-3-319-08391-9   ISBN 978-3-319-08392-6 (eBook)
DOI 10.1007/978-3-319-08392-6
Springer Cham Heidelberg New York Dordrecht London

Library of Congress Control Number: 2014944438

Printed on acid-free paper

Springer is part of Springer Science+Business Media (www.springer.com)

Preface

This book evolved from parts of the first author's dissertation and aims to give an overview of state-of-the-art approaches to motion estimation and motion correction in positron emission tomography (PET) – and even going one step beyond. Besides these central topics, we provide some general information for all related topics, such as the principle of PET or gating. However, in order not to lose focus we do not go into too much details. Interested readers are referred to further literature regarding these topics.

This book is aimed at all those working in the field of (thoracic) PET imaging. While the book is rather written from a methodological perspective, it also provides a general overview over the topic of motion estimation and motion correction. Hence, also more practically oriented people will benefit from reading it, while skipping the theoretical parts.

Writing this book was only possible due to the great support of various colleagues. A particular thanks goes to all our colleagues at the European Institute for Molecular Imaging (EIMI, head: Prof. Michael Schäfers). In particular, thanks goes to Thomas Kösters for providing his reconstruction software EMRECON and to Florian Büther for providing his list mode driven gating software.

The VAMPIRE approach and the accompanied advancements were developed in collaboration with Martin Burger, Jan Modersitzki, Lars Ruthotto, and Carsten H. Wolters. Especially, we thank Jan Modersitzki for his advice regarding the implementation, nice discussions, and for making his FAIR image registration toolbox freely available. Thanks goes to Christoph Brune with whom the mass-preserving optical flow approach was developed. Further, a deep thanks goes to Lars Ruthotto for fruitful discussions and proofreading.

Finally, we thank the Department of Nuclear Medicine, University Hospital of Münster, who helped with the acquisition of the human PET list mode data. This work was partly funded by the Deutsche Forschungsgemeinschaft, SFB 656 MoBil (projects B2 and B3).

Münster, Germany   Fabian Gigengack
April 2014   Xiaoyi Jiang
                                                              Mohammad Dawood
                                                              Klaus P. Schäfers

Contents

Acronyms

^{18}F-FDG	Fluorodeoxyglucose.
AC	Attenuation correction.
ACF	Attenuation coefficient factor.
CT	Computed tomography.
ECG	Electrocardiogram.
FAIR	Flexible Algorithms for Image Registration.
FOV	Field of view.
FWHM	Full width half maximum.
HLA	Horizontal long axis.
LOR	Line of response.
MCIR	Motion compensated image reconstruction.
MLAA	Maximum likelihood reconstruction of attenuation and activity.
MPOF	Mass-preserving optical flow.
MRI	Magnetic resonance imaging.
NAC	Non-attenuation corrected.
NCC	Normalized cross-correlation.
PET	Positron emission tomography.
PSF	Point spread function.
PVE	Partial volume effect.
SA	Short axis.
SAD	Sum of absolute differences.
SNR	Signal-to-noise-ratio.
SPECT	Single photon emission computed tomography.
SSD	Sum of squared differences.
TOF	Time-of-flight.
VAMPIRE	Variational Algorithm for Mass-Preserving Image REgistration.
VLA	Vertical long axis.

Notation

$\mathbb{R}^d$ d-dimensional Euclidean space of real numbers with the Euclidean norm $|\cdot|$.

$\boldsymbol{x}$ Point $\boldsymbol{x} = (x,y,z)^T \in \mathbb{R}^3$.

$|\cdot|$ Euclidean norm (or L_2 norm) in $\mathbb{R}^3$, i.e., $|\boldsymbol{x}| := \sqrt{x^2+y^2+z^2}$.

$|X|$ For a set $X \subset \mathbb{R}^3$ the notation $|\cdot|$ denotes $|X| := \int_X d\boldsymbol{x}$.

Ω Image domain $\Omega \subset \mathbb{R}^3$.

$\mathcal{I}$ Image sequence $\mathcal{I} : \Omega \times \mathbb{R} \to \mathbb{R}$.

$\mathcal{T}$ Template image $\mathcal{T} : \Omega \to \mathbb{R}$.

$\mathcal{R}$ Reference image $\mathcal{R} : \Omega \to \mathbb{R}$.

$\mathcal{T}_r^c$ Template image in dual gating with respiratory phase r and cardiac phase c.

$\boldsymbol{y}$ Transformation $\boldsymbol{y} : \mathbb{R}^3 \to \mathbb{R}^3$ with $\boldsymbol{y}(\boldsymbol{x}) = \boldsymbol{x} + \boldsymbol{u}(\boldsymbol{x})$, $\boldsymbol{x} \in \mathbb{R}^3$.

$\boldsymbol{u}$ Deformation $\boldsymbol{u} : \mathbb{R}^3 \to \mathbb{R}^3$ with $\boldsymbol{u}(\boldsymbol{x}) = \boldsymbol{y}(\boldsymbol{x}) - \boldsymbol{x}$, $\boldsymbol{x} \in \mathbb{R}^3$.

$\boldsymbol{y}_p$ Parametric transformation $\boldsymbol{y}_p : \mathbb{R}^3 \to \mathbb{R}^3$ based on parameter vector p.

$\mathcal{I}_i$ $\mathcal{I}_i := \frac{\partial}{\partial i}\mathcal{I}$ is the partial derivative of $\mathcal{I}$ with respect to the variable i, $i = x,y,z$.

$\mathcal{I}_{i,j}$ $\mathcal{I}_{i,j} := \frac{\partial^2}{\partial i \partial j}\mathcal{I}$ is the second-order partial derivative of $\mathcal{I}$ with $i,j = x,y,z$.

$\nabla\mathcal{I}$ $\nabla\mathcal{I} := (\mathcal{I}_x, \mathcal{I}_y, \mathcal{I}_z)^T$ are the partial derivatives of $\mathcal{I}$.

$\nabla\boldsymbol{y}$ Jacobian matrix of the transformation $\boldsymbol{y}$.

$\nabla \cdot \mathcal{I}$ Divergence of $\mathcal{I}$ defined by $\nabla \cdot \mathcal{I} := \mathcal{I}_x + \mathcal{I}_y + \mathcal{I}_z$.

Cof   Cofactor matrix.

det   Determinant.

$\Delta\mathcal{I}$ Laplacian of $\mathcal{I}$ defined by $\Delta\mathcal{I} := \mathcal{I}_{x,x} + \mathcal{I}_{y,y} + \mathcal{I}_{z,z}$.

$\mathcal{D}$ Distance term.

$\mathcal{S}$ Regularization term.

$\mathcal{J}$ Registration functional – usually of the form $\mathcal{J} = \mathcal{D} + \alpha \cdot \mathcal{S}$.

α Scalar weighting factor $\alpha \in \mathbb{R}^{>0}$.

$\mathcal{M}$ Transformation model, e.g., standard model $\mathcal{M}^{\text{std}}(\mathcal{T}, \boldsymbol{y}) := \mathcal{T} \circ \boldsymbol{y}$.

e Average endpoint error $e(\boldsymbol{y}_1, \boldsymbol{y}_2) := \frac{1}{|\Omega|} \int_\Omega |\boldsymbol{y}_1(\boldsymbol{x}) - \boldsymbol{y}_2(\boldsymbol{x})| d\boldsymbol{x}$.

$e^{\max}$ Maximum endpoint error $e^{\max}(\boldsymbol{y}_1, \boldsymbol{y}_2) := \max_{\boldsymbol{x} \in \Omega} |\boldsymbol{y}_1(\boldsymbol{x}) - \boldsymbol{y}_2(\boldsymbol{x})|$.

Chapter 1
Introduction

Molecular imaging is gaining more and more importance, particularly Positron Emission Tomography (PET) being the tomographic modality with the highest molecular sensitivity. However, motion is a known problem for many medical imaging modalities that require a minimum acquisition time to collect the relevant information for image generation. Emission tomography techniques, such as PET or Single Photon Emission Computed Tomography (SPECT) are particularly affected by motion since respiratory and cardiac motion lead to image degradation in thoracic studies. Image blurring and wrong attenuation correction are possible unwanted consequences which can impair clinical diagnosis.

The aim of this chapter is to provide insight into the backgrounds necessary for motion estimation and motion correction in PET. This includes an introduction to the modality PET itself, gating, and effects which impair image quality, i.e., Partial Volume Effects (PVE). This chapter concludes with an overview of state-of-the-art literature regarding motion estimation respectively motion correction.

1.1 Motivation

Both respiratory and cardiac motion are sources of degradation in thoracic PET since the PET images are acquired over an elongated period of time (in the range of minutes). During this acquisition time lung and heart motion occurs which leads to imaging artifacts: wrong attenuation correction and image blur. Attenuation correction is the method of correcting the PET data for the effects of photon absorption in the body. Dense tissues like bones absorb a larger part of the photons than less dense tissues like lungs. Therefore, PET images without attenuation correction show apparently greater activity in areas with less density. This effect is corrected by scaling the number of photons registered in the PET scanner in accordance with the density of tissues. When using Computed Tomography (CT) for

© The Author(s) 2015
F. Gigengack et al., *Motion Correction in Thoracic Positron Emission Tomography*,
SpringerBriefs in Electrical and Computer Engineering,
DOI 10.1007/978-3-319-08392-6_1

attenuation correction, the CT images themselves hardly suffer from motion since they are usually acquired during breath holding and can be corrected for cardiac motion by prospective electrocardiogram (ECG) triggering. In the presence of severe motion, however, part of the PET data may not be in spatial correspondence with the CT data and will be wrongly corrected for attenuation, e.g., activity from the heart may be corrected with lung density [11, 34, 56, 105, 106], cf. Fig. 2.13.

Another unwanted effect of motion is image blur. Motion at the source of radioactive emission results in a spatial blurring in the reconstructed PET images proportional to the magnitude of motion and thus loss of contrast. Generally, the inherent motion during PET image acquisition has a number of negative consequences like wrong attenuation correction (see above), misstaging of tumors [42], inaccurate localization of lesions [105], and wrong calculation of standard uptake values [96]. Therefore, there is a strong need of reducing motion artifacts for advanced PET imaging.

Gating-based techniques were found applicable for this purpose [87]. Gating is the decomposition of the whole data set into units that represent different breathing and/or cardiac phases [23], cf. Sect. 1.3. After gating, each single gate shows little motion only, but suffers from a relatively low Signal-to-Noise-Ratio (SNR) and a reduced contrast as only a small portion of all available events is used [133]. The fact that images contain both cardiac and respiratory motion motivates the reduction of both types by means of dual gating introduced in Sect. 1.3.3. Most approaches in the literature deal with respiratory motion only. However, as maximal displacements for cardiac motion of 42 mm [134] are in the same range as maximal respiratory displacements of 23 mm [122], the cardiac motion component should be treated as well.

The effect of motion and gating is demonstrated in Fig. 1.1 with cardiac planes of a human heart (20 min ^{18}F-FDG PET scan without attenuation correction). An introduction to the used visualizations is given in Sect. 1.6. A reconstruction of the whole data set without gating can be seen in Fig. 1.1a. Respiratory and cardiac motion causes an obvious blurring of the heart contour. In contrast, a single phase of the respiratory and cardiac cycle (dual gating with five respiratory and five cardiac gates) is shown in Fig. 1.1b. The blurring is clearly reduced. However, simultaneously the amount of noise is increased due to the reduced number of events used for the reconstruction. Furthermore, motion leads to an apparently higher blood pool activity in the image without gating compared to the other images. This phenomenon is illustrated with line profiles in Fig. 1.1d. The left plot shows the line profiles of the first column from left to right (respectively the second column from left to right). The middle plot shows the line profiles of the first column from top to bottom (respectively the third column from top to bottom). The right plot shows the line profiles of the second column from bottom to top (respectively the third column from left to right). The maximum peaks of the dotted profile (no gating) are clearly lower in the central plot compared to the dashed profile (single gate). The overall aim of gating-based motion correction is to combine the reduced blurring achieved by gating in Fig. 1.1b with the full statistics of the whole measurement in Fig. 1.1a towards enhanced motion compensated PET images. A preview of the result after applying our proposed methods is finally given in Fig. 1.1c.

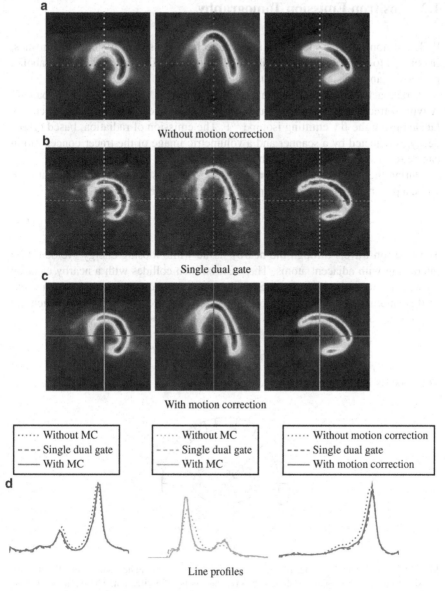

Fig. 1.1 (a) Slices of the cardiac axes of a reconstruction using the whole acquired PET data, (b) one single respiratory and cardiac phase, and (c) after Motion Correction (MC). The image with MC (using our VAMPIRE method) combines the advantages of the above images: reduced motion artifacts and a low noise level. Line profiles are given in (d)

1.2   Positron Emission Tomography

PET is a non-invasive molecular imaging technique used in medical diagnostics. In contrast to morphological imaging modalities like CT, functional, i.e., metabolic, processes can be visualized and quantified.

A radioactively labeled substance called *tracer* is administered to a patient. A typical tracer is Fluorodeoxyglucose (^{18}F-FDG) where glucose is radioactively labeled using the β^+ emitting isotope ^{18}F. The emission of radiation, based on β^+ decay, is detected by a scanner and a volumetric image of the tracer concentration can be reconstructed to visualize the metabolism.

During the β^+ decay of a ^{18}F nucleus a proton p is converted into a neutron n while a positron e^+ and an electron neutrino v_e is emitted

$$p \rightarrow n + e^+ + v_e \,. \tag{1.1}$$

The positron travels through the nearby tissue while loosing energy (velocity) by interacting with adjacent atoms. The positron then collides with a nearby electron e^- which is its antiparticle, having the same mass, but opposite charge. As a result of this annihilation, two gamma photons γ are produced with 511 keV which are emitted approximately in opposite directions (angle of $\sim 180°$)

$$e^+ + e^- \rightarrow 2\gamma \,. \tag{1.2}$$

This process is illustrated in Fig. 1.2.

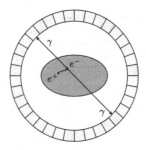

Fig. 1.2 As a result of β^+ decay, the emitted positron e^+ annihilates with a nearby electron e^- which results in two gamma photons γ traveling in opposite direction. These photons can be recorded by detectors, circularly arranged around the patient. The length of the path of the positron to the electron (positron range, see Sect. 1.4.2) is rather short with about 0.1 mm Full Width Half Maximum (FWHM) [109]

The architecture of most PET scanners is based on circularly arranged detector blocks, see Fig. 1.2. Each detector block consists of a certain number of single detectors elements. To increase the Field Of View (FOV) and the sensitivity of the scanner, several detector rings are usually stacked together.

If a single gamma photon (within a pre-defined energy window) is detected by the scanner, a short time window of a few nanoseconds (ns) is opened. A photon arriving at an opposite detector within this time window is assumed to be the corresponding partner photon originating from the same annihilation process. In this case we speak of a *coincidence*. It is assumed that the underlying radioactive decay has its origin somewhere on the line connecting these two detectors. This idea forms the basis for image reconstruction where these lines are called *Lines Of Response* (LOR).

The acquisition mode in PET can either be list mode or sinogram mode. In list mode acquisition, the coincidences that are detected by the PET scanner are written into a list. Each list item contains a time tag and the detector pair that registered the coincidence. For many reconstruction techniques, the list is processed in a rebinning step to a so called sinogram (line-integral data). The sorting of the sinograms is based on the angle of each view and tilt. In sinogram mode acquisition, the sinogram data is computed directly without outputting the list mode data.

Based on a huge number of these coincidences it is possible to reconstruct a 3D image volume. During this reconstruction process, various physical effects (e.g., photon attenuation, photon scattering, randomly detected coincidences, etc.) can be accounted for and dedicated corrections can be applied. Ideally, the underlying radioactivity concentration can be derived from the images in absolute numbers making PET to a unique non-invasive imaging technique.

All reconstructions throughout this book were made with the EM reconstruction software EMRECON [77, 78] which is a representative of the discrete (3D) EM reconstruction framework. The implementation is based on the standard MLEM [124] and OS-MLEM [65] methods.

1.3 Gating of PET Data

We have seen in Sect. 1.1 that the quality of PET images is corrupted by inherent cardiac and respiratory motion. A common approach to reduce motion artifacts is to perform so-called *gating*. The basic idea of gating is to divide the list mode stream into small units according to the different motion phases. Each of the small units contains only measured data which belongs to the corresponding motion phase. Subsequently the image of each individual motion phase is reconstructed.

As a consequence, the amount of motion in each image is reduced to a minimum. However, the motion reduction comes along with a simultaneous reduction of statistics. An unwanted increase in the noise level and a reduced image contrast is the result [133]. The problem of increased noise and reduced contrast can be overcome by motion correction techniques, as discussed in this book. The basic idea of these techniques is to estimate motion between the different motion phases and correct for it, which finally allows to use all available list mode information for the motion corrected image.

Gating techniques are based on list mode streams (cf. Sect. 1.2) which particularly provide information about the exact time of detection for each coincidence.

If a synchronized motion signal (e.g., respiratory and/or cardiac) is recorded simultaneously to the PET measurement, each event can be assigned a particular motion phase. The fraction of events belonging to only one of these motion phases can then be used to reconstruct an image, representing the particular motion phase, which we call *gate*.

The prerequisite for gating is thus the extraction of motion information in terms of a gating signal. This can either be done *extrinsically* or *intrinsically*. Extrinsically means that the actual motion is derived from external measurable correlated motion. Intrinsically means that the actual motion itself is measured. Examples for the acquisition of the gating signal are given for respiratory and cardiac gating in Sects. 1.3.1 and 1.3.2.

The subdivision or binning of the gating signal can be performed

- *Amplitude-based* (Example in Fig. 1.3) or
- *Phase-based* (Example in Fig. 1.5),

whereas each method can either be with

- Equal widths or
- Variable widths

throughout all cycles. For variable widths the division can again either be with

- Equal widths within each cycle or
- Variable widths within each cycle.

For more details about this classification, including illustrations, we refer to [32,35].

Specific information about the individual gating schemes for *respiratory* and *cardiac* motion are summarized in Sects. 1.3.1 and 1.3.2. We will further derive the combination of both gating schemes, entitled *dual gating*, in Sect. 1.3.3. More information regarding gating is also given in Chap. 4 where possible future advances and developments in the field of PET motion correction are discussed.

1.3.1 Respiratory Gating

The correction of respiratory motion is considered primarily in the literature of thoracic PET as respiration can lead to attenuation induced artifacts, cf. Sect. 1.1. The objective of *respiratory gating* is thus to create a set of images that represent the different motion phases of respiration, going from expiration to inspiration or vice versa. To allow a partition of the list mode stream, a synchronized respiratory signal is needed for the PET measurement.

Extrinsic devices [34, 98] (like pressure sensor, spirometer, temperature sensor, external markers, camera devices) are commonly used to obtain the respiratory signal. A monotonic correlation of the extrinsically obtained signal to the breathing motion is assumed. In practice, this assumption is approximately valid [67, 116].

Recently, intrinsic data driven gating schemes have been investigated as they do not require any extra effort at the time of the scan in terms of auxiliary measurements [23]. The respiratory signal is estimated on basis of list mode data itself. To this end, the list mode stream is divided into small time frames (about 50 ms [23]) with subsequent computation of the axial center of mass along the scanner axis of the measured counting rates in the respective frames. The respiratory signal can then be deduced from changes in the center of mass.

The illustration of an amplitude-based respiratory gating scheme with variable widths and equal widths within each cycle is shown in Fig. 1.3. This scheme was found to be superior to other gating schemes [35].

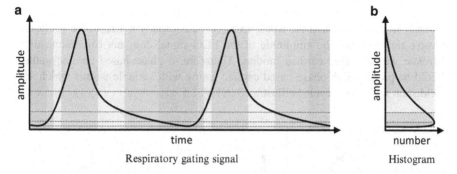

Fig. 1.3 The respiratory signal (*solid black curve* in (**a**)) is processed into a histogram in (**b**). The amplitude is divided into sections (*vertical sections* in (**b**)) with variable widths such that each section has the same area under the curve of the histogram. The amplitude subdivision remains constant throughout all cycles. This subdivision is transferred back to the respiratory gating signal which is then divided into different temporal sections (*horizontal sections* in (**a**)). All sections belonging to the same vertical section in (**b**) together represent one of the respiratory gates

An example of respiratory gating applied to patient data can be seen in Fig. 1.4. The list mode data set was divided into four gates according to an amplitude-based respiratory gating scheme with variable widths and equal widths within each cycle, cf. Fig. 1.3. More gates, typically in the range of eight to ten gates, are used in practice [36].

1.3.2 Cardiac Gating

The objective of *cardiac gating* is to create a set of images that represent the different motion phases of the cardiac cycle, going from diastole over systole back to diastole. For capturing the cardiac motion, a triggered ECG file can be recorded (synchronized) to the PET scan. Usually only the R-wave time points are stored. Based on this information a phase-based subdivision can be performed with equidistant or variable intervals.

Respiratory gate 1   Respiratory gate 2   Respiratory gate 3   Respiratory gate 4
(expiration)   (inspiration)

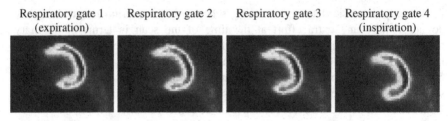

Fig. 1.4 The amplitude-based respiratory gating scheme in Fig. 1.3 was applied to patient data (20 min ^{18}F-FDG PET scan without attenuation correction). The respiratory signal was extracted with the data driven method proposed in [23]. The images show coronal slices of the left ventricle going from expiration to inspiration. The axial (up-down) motion is clearly visible

Apart from the fact that the *whole* ECG curve is usually not recorded (only the R-wave time points), the amplitude of the ECG signal does not (monotonically) correlate with the true cardiac motion. Therefore, a phase-based cardiac gating should be preferred. A phase-based cardiac gating with variable widths which are equidistant within one cycle is illustrated in Fig. 1.5.

Fig. 1.5 An ECG signal (*solid curve*) is divided into variable sections which are equidistant within one cycle. The totality of all corresponding sections represent a single cardiac gate

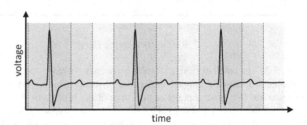

An example of cardiac gating applied to patient data can be found in Fig. 1.6. The list mode data set was divided into four gates according to an phase-based cardiac gating with variable widths which are equidistant within one cycle, cf. Fig. 1.5. Similarly to respiratory gating, more gates (about ten gates) are typically used in practice.

Cardiac gate 1   Cardiac gate 2   Cardiac gate 3   Cardiac gate 4
(end-systole)   (end-diastole)

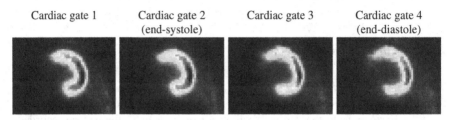

Fig. 1.6 The phase-based cardiac gating in Fig. 1.5 was applied to patient data (20 min ^{18}F-FDG PET scan without attenuation correction). The R-wave time points of an ECG signal were used to perform cardiac gating. The images show coronal slices of the left ventricle going from diastole over systole back to diastole. The contraction of the heart is clearly visible

Cardiac motion is hitherto rarely considered in methods for motion correction. It poses new challenges to motion correction techniques due to partial volume effect (see Sect. 1.4) induced intensity modulations. This issue is addressed and resolved in Chap. 2 (Sect. 2.1.4 respectively Sect. 2.2.4) as one of the major contributions of this book.

1.3.3 Dual Gating

In pure respiratory gated PET, each gate still contains cardiac motion. Analogously, pure cardiac gated PET images still contain respiratory motion. This can be observed in Figs. 1.4 and 1.6. *Dual gating* is an attempt to even further reduce the amount of motion contained in the images [74, 76, 81, 82, 92, 127]. In dual gating, an $n \times m$ matrix of n cardiac and m respiratory images is built, i.e., each cardiac phase is over again divided into all respiratory phases (or vice versa). Consequently, time information about cardiac and respiratory motion is required. Options for the division of the individual components of motion are discussed in the above Sects. 1.3.1 and 1.3.2. For a more detailed explanation of dual gating we refer to [92].

The same patient data used for the pure respiratory and pure cardiac gating in Figs. 1.4 and 1.6 serves as the basis for the 4×4 dual gating shown in Fig. 1.7. It can be seen that dual gating features an increased reduction of motion artifacts compared to pure respiratory or pure cardiac gating. This is, of course, accompanied by increased noise levels. Techniques to overcome the noise problem are provided in Sect. 3.2 with a simplified pipeline for motion correction.

1.4 Partial Volume Effect and Mass-Preservation

The basic principles of the PET image generation process were already introduced in Sect. 1.2. In this section we will discuss some further properties of this process, known as the Partial Volume Effect (PVE), which lead to a loss of spatial resolution. The PVE can be divided into two distinct components:

1. Tissue fraction (Sect. 1.4.1) and
2. Spill-over (Sect. 1.4.2).

Especially in cardiac gated PET (cf. Sect. 1.3.2), the PVE can lead to varying intensities at corresponding anatomical points in different gates (cf. Fig. 1.11), which impairs motion estimation. The identification of the radioactivity-preservation principle (respectively mass-preservation) in Sect. 1.4.3 allows to account for this effect during motion estimation.

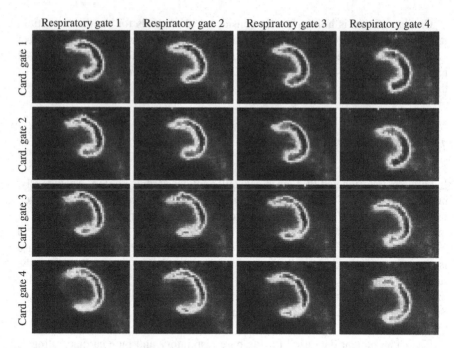

Fig. 1.7 Example of a 4×4 dual gating of patient data. The images show coronal slices of the left ventricle. The rows vary in the cardiac and the columns in the respiratory phases. The respiratory and cardiac gating signal was determined as described in connection with Figs. 1.4 and 1.6

1.4.1   PVE: Tissue Fraction

One component of the PVE, called *tissue fraction*, results from the discretization of the measured data on a finite voxel grid. The intensity value of a voxel is given by an averaging of all measured data inside the volume defined by the voxel.

Figure 1.8 illustrates tissue fraction at the borderline of two neighboring "tissues" in a 1D example. The signal with tissue fraction shows mixed intensities at the border of neighboring structures (in this case of the zero background and the foreground peak). These averaged intensities, however, do not appear in the original signal.

1.4.2   PVE: Spill-Over

During the process of PET data acquisition, several factors lead to image degradation. Suppose a point source is measured, the reconstructed image would show a smeared-out version of the original signal. The signal of the point source is spilled

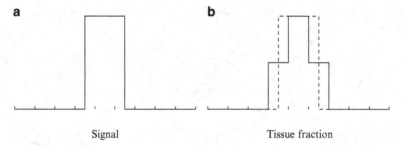

Fig. 1.8 Tissue fraction for a 1D signal. Tics on x-axis denote sampling intervals. (**a**) Input signal. (**b**) Due to tissue fraction the signal is an average of the intensities within each respective sampling area. The input signal is plotted as a *dashed line* in (**b**) for orientation

over to the neighborhood which is why we speak of the *spill-over* effect. This effect and the combination of spill-over and tissue fraction is illustrated in a 1D example in Fig. 1.9.

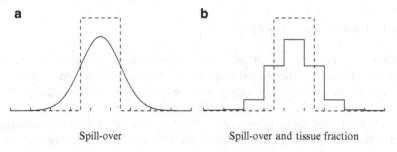

Fig. 1.9 Partial volume effects for the 1D input signal given in Fig. 1.8a. Tics on x-axis denote sampling intervals. (**a**) Spill-over causes part of the signal intensity to appear outside of the peak area. (**b**) Combined effect of tissue fraction and spill-over. The input signal is plotted as a *dashed line* for orientation

The spill-over effect can be thought of as a convolution of the original signal with a (locally adaptive) filter mask. The filter mask is called *Point Spread Function* (PSF) and is often approximated by a Gaussian kernel. The disruptive factors which are responsible for the spill-over effect in PET are illustrated in Fig. 1.10 and will be described in more detail in the following.

1.4.2.1 Positron Range

In β^+ decay, the emitted positron travels a short path until it annihilates with an electron. This distance is called the *positron range* and complicates the exact

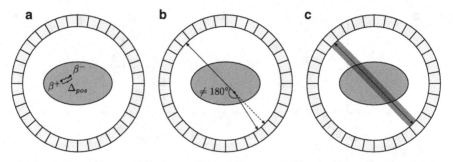

Fig. 1.10 The spill-over effect is caused by various errors which impair the exact spatial localization of measured coincidences. (**a**) Positron range Δ_{pos}. (**b**) Photon non-collinearity. (**c**) Detector width

localization of the event's origin. See Fig. 1.10a for an illustration of the positron range. The positron range for a typical tracer like ^{18}F-FDG results in a blurring of about 0.1 mm FWHM [109] in the resulting image.

1.4.2.2   Photon Non-collinearity

The two gamma photons which result from the annihilation process fly in opposite directions. However, if the annihilating particles have a remaining momentum, the angle can deviate from 180°, resulting in a *non-collinearity* of the gamma photons. The dashed line in the illustration in Fig. 1.10b hints the supposed path of the photon. The actual detection, however, takes place at a different location, indicated by the solid line. The photon non-collinearity for ^{18}F results in a blurring of about $d \cdot 0.0022$ FWHM [109] (in the center of the scanner), where d (in mm) is the diameter of the scanner.

1.4.2.3   Detector Width

Even assuming the previous factors were not present, the events measured in the volume connecting a detector pair can only be localized with an accuracy down to (half) the *detector width*. All coincidences measured by a certain detector pair are treated as if they had taken place in the very center of the detector. All coincidences between the detector pair connected by the gray area in Fig. 1.10c which occurred in this gray area are virtually positioned at the center line connecting the detector pair. This is indicated by the solid line. Given a detector width of w, a blurring of about $w/2$ FWHM results in the center of the scanner.

1.4.3 Mass-Preservation

Tissue compression and PVE, as introduced in Sects. 1.4.1 and 1.4.2, lead to intensity modulations at corresponding points in different gated reconstructions [91]. Especially for relatively thin structures like the myocardium the true uptake values are affected by the PVE. A patient example is given in Fig. 1.11 where a systolic and diastolic slice (same respiratory phase) and corresponding line profiles of a dual gated 3D data set are shown. Especially the maximum intensity values of the two heart phases indicate that corresponding points can differ in intensity.

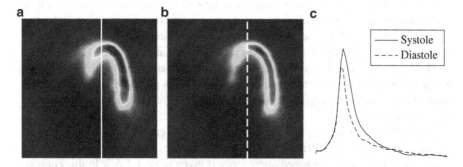

Fig. 1.11 Slices of the HLA (cf. Sect. 1.6) of the (**a**) systole and (**b**) diastole and (**c**) corresponding line profiles for patient data. The *solid line* belongs to the systole and the *dashed line* to the diastole. It can be observed that the maximum peaks in these line profiles vary a lot due to the PVE

To deal with the challenges caused by intensity artifacts, we consider the mass-preserving property of PET images. In gating, all gates are formed over the same time interval, i.e., the whole acquisition time. Hence, the total amount of radioactivity in each gate is approximately equal. In other words, in any respiratory and/or cardiac gate no radioactivity can be lost or added apart from some minor changes at the edges of the field of view. We refer to this property as *mass-preservation* in the following.

To further illustrate the mass-preserving property we artificially construct two 2D structures with different width and height in Fig. 1.12 and simulate the PVE as performed in connection with Fig. 1.9b. The integral over the total intensity (respectively mass) of the two signals is equal. The original signals are shown in the top row of Fig. 1.12. The same signals with simulated PVE are shown in the mid row. Line profiles through the images, shown in the bottom row, illustrate the varying intensities after simulating the PVE (solid lines) compared to the original images with the same maximal intensity (dashed line).

1.5   Introduction to Motion Correction

The objective of this section is to provide an overview of the most important topics related to motion correction for thoracic PET. Several approaches were proposed recently to reduce motion and its effects on further analysis. Apart from simple or optimized PET gating procedures, most PET motion correction schemes are either based on a two-step approach (motion estimation followed by motion correction) or try to correct for motion in a combined estimation/correction algorithm. Motion estimation/correction approaches can be divided into *intrinsic*, *extrinsic*, and *hybrid* methods which are discussed in Sect. 1.5.1.

With intrinsic we refer to approaches where motion is estimated on the PET data itself. In extrinsic approaches motion is derived from an additional accompanying measurement. Hybrid approaches represent a combination of intrinsic and extrinsic approaches, taking advantage of the PET as well as the auxiliary data.

One can also characterize the various motion estimation methods based on the way how the motion is technically estimated. From this perspective, two classes of methods, namely *image registration* and *optical flow*, are dominating in the current literature, cf. Sect. 1.5.2.

As we have seen in the previous Section, mass-preserving motion estimation is of essential importance when working with PET images. A taxonomy with related work of *mass-preservation* based approaches is given in Sect. 1.5.3. In this context, *diffeomorphic* transformations are imperative for medical image registration. This aspect of motion estimation will be discussed in Sect. 1.5.4.

1.5.1   Intrinsic vs. Extrinsic Methods

1.5.1.1   Intrinsic Approaches

In most approaches motion is estimated intrinsically on the basis of the PET data itself. They can be classified into four groups according to [8, 51]:

- Averaging of aligned images [8, 34, 51, 73],
- Re-reconstruction using a time-varying system matrix [46, 80, 111, 112],
- Event rebinning [79],
- Joint reconstruction of image and motion [12, 13, 20, 68, 89, 121].

For more information and literature about the four groups we refer to Sect. 3.1.

1.5.1.2   Extrinsic Approaches

Based on PET data alone, adequate motion estimates can only be expected in regions of sufficient tracer uptake. Hence, additional *extrinsic* motion sources, such

Fig. 1.12 The original signals in the *top row* are blurred with a Gaussian kernel to simulate the spill-over effect of the PVE, which is shown in the *mid row*. The tissue fraction effect is clearly visible in terms of the discretization. Line profiles through these images, indicated by the *solid* and *dashed lines*, are shown in the *bottom row*. The *dashed lines* of the original signals reach the same maximum intensity. The *solid lines* show a discrepancy in the maximum values, which makes brightness constancy based registration approaches inapplicable

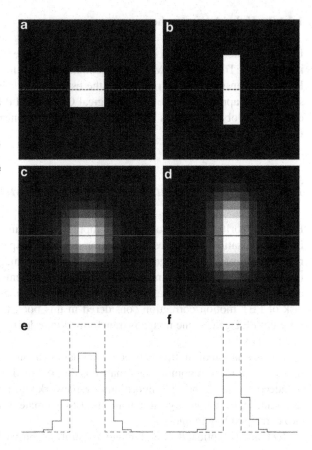

as Magnetic Resonance Imaging (MRI) or CT data, are increasingly used in recent publications (see also the discussion in Sect. 4.4). Approaches using data from combined PET/CT or PET/MRI scanners were investigated by estimating the motion fields based on the morphological CT [80, 84, 111] or MRI [29, 39, 44, 45, 58, 108] data and applying them subsequently to the sequentially or even simultaneously acquired PET data. The methods sound promising as they are capable of providing accurate motion information even for regions which show no high uptake in the PET images (e.g., small lesions). To keep the radiation burden for the patient as small as possible, recent approaches are based on MRI data and refrain from using CT acquisitions. However, combined PET/MRI systems are not yet available everywhere and, among other things, the MRI acquisition protocols for respiratory gating are still under development.

1.5.1.3 Hybrid Approaches

In extrinsic methods motion is estimated using solely the CT or MRI data. However, in case of PET/CT or PET/MRI data from all available image sources, i.e., also the PET data, can make a contribution to the estimation of the underlying motion. In such *hybrid* approaches, the morphological CT or MRI data will guide the motion estimation globally whereas PET can have a valuable contribution in regions of high tracer uptake [43,53].

1.5.2 Image Registration vs. Optical Flow Methods

From an algorithmic point of view the motion in PET images can be estimated by image registration techniques. Registration denotes the spatial alignment of two corresponding images. In the general context of medical imaging these corresponding images can be obtained from the same or different patients, acquired at the same or at a different time, using the same or different scanning techniques. For the special task of PET motion correction considered in this book these images are given as different PET gates. One image is transformed in order to match the other image as good as possible.

The estimation of motion between two images can not only be done by means of image registration. A common alternative is the so-called optical flow. The objective is indeed the same, but the algorithmic framework and actual implementation are different. Optical flow algorithms are used to estimate a dense flow field between two corresponding images.

Technically, optical flow and image registration approaches provide significantly different approaches to motion estimation. In this book we will follow both paths of motion estimation in Chap. 2, in particular their mass-preserving versions. A comparison of the two approaches will be given in Sect. 2.3.

1.5.3 Mass-Preserving Motion Estimation

In the general literature on motion estimation the intensity modulation problem is hardly considered. Even in medical imaging most of the existing approaches do not deal with it explicitly as they focus mainly on respiratory motion correction where intensity modulation is of less importance. In the following we briefly discuss mass-preserving transformation models that were already applied to different kinds of medical data. Generally speaking, mass-preserving image registration is the correct model for data that represent densities as in the case of PET, SPECT, and CT.

1.5.3.1   CT

The compressibility of the lungs makes motion estimation in CT lung images challenging. A mass-preserving registration framework was applied to such data in [138] to compensate for tissue compression. The proposed multi-resolution B-spline approach includes an essential additional mapping of the Hounsfield units to density values. A similar approach for CT lung registration is proposed in [57].

1.5.3.2   MRI

Field inhomogeneities lead to image degradation in MRI, particularly in Echo Planar Imaging (EPI) sequences. Mislocalizations along the read-out direction are successfully corrected with a mass-preserving transformation model in [27, 104, 118]. A peculiarity of the proposed method is the simultaneous application of the same transformation to two corresponding reference scans but with reversed direction.

1.5.3.3   SPECT

The expansion ratio characterizes the ratio of volume change of the heart in cardiac SPECT. In order to achieve the preservation of the overall radioactivity the expansion ratio was incorporated into the objective function for motion estimation in [91, 129] by rescaling the pixel intensity in accordance with the wall thickening. The proposed deformable mesh model is based on a left-ventricle surface model.

1.5.3.4   PET

For PET, we proposed two approaches for mass-preserving motion estimation with the Variational Algorithm for Mass-Preserving Image REgistration (VAMPIRE) [50, 51] and the Mass-Preserving Optical Flow (MPOF) approach [33,37]. Both methods compensate for tissue compression and, more importantly, allow the matching of corresponding points with PVE disturbed intensities. The second property distinguishes the application of mass-preserving motion estimation methods to PET data compared to CT or MRI. Note, however, that these methods could also be applied to SPECT data for the same reasons.

VAMPIRE and MPOF account for the preservation of mass with a specifically designed transformation model considering the volume change induced by the estimated transformation. The same effect could also be achieved by utilizing a forward mapping as proposed by Klein [71, 72]. However, as such a transformation model is not necessarily surjective, a sampling of each point in the reference domain is not guaranteed. Furthermore, a complicated energy function with numerous local minima due to the forward deformation mapping is reported by Klein. Because of these drawbacks, we do not consider such methods based on forward mapping in the following.

1.5.4 Diffeomorphic Registration

In medical image registration, diffeomorphic transformations are imperative as they are invertible, smooth, orientation preserving, and free of foldings. Recently, several approaches were developed to ensure diffeomorphisms [2, 5, 97, 117, 132]. Inspired by the Jacobian determinant in VAMPIRE, we derived a new discretization of a hyperelastic regularizer [22] that is now integrated in the FAIR registration tool-box [95]. It directly controls the volumetric change which in our case corresponds to the intensity modulations. Although it is a key feature of VAMPIRE, it can also be used for any other registration task. The main ideas of this regularizer are summarized in Sect. 2.1.2.3.

1.6 Visualization

For the illustration of the data we will use two different visualizations in terms of *body planes* and *cardiac planes*. To better understand their location with respect to the patient they will be introduced briefly below. The global body planes are

1. *Sagittal,*
2. *Coronal,* and
3. *Transverse.*

The transverse plane is also often denoted as the *axial plane* in the literature. An illustration is given in Fig. 1.13.

Apart from the global body planes we will also use cardiac planes which are given by the

1. *Short Axis* (SA),
2. *Horizontal Long Axis* (HLA), and the
3. *Vertical Long Axis* (VLA).

The cardiac planes are visualized in Fig. 1.14. The cardiac planes are especially informative for physicians as they are given in the coordinate system of the heart. However, as for example respiratory motion is primarily in the craniocaudal direction, which can be nicely visualized by the coronal or sagittal plane, we will use all representations throughout this book.

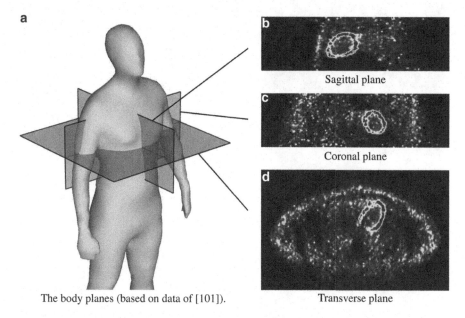

The body planes (based on data of [101]).   Transverse plane

Fig. 1.13 Illustration of the three body planes: sagittal, coronal, and transverse. The location of the planes relative to the patient are illustrated in (**a**). Example images for the thoracic region are shown in (**b**)–(**d**)

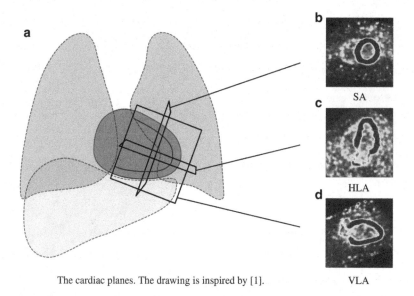

The cardiac planes. The drawing is inspired by [1].   VLA

Fig. 1.14 Illustration of the three cardiac planes: SA, HLA, and VLA. The location of the planes relative to the patient are illustrated in (**a**). Example images for the heart are shown in (**b**)–(**d**)

Chapter 2
Motion Estimation

In the introduction of this book we have seen that PET image acquisition is suscep-
tible to motion artifacts. The first step to overcome this problem is the separation of
the measured data into different motion states via gating as described in Sect. 1.3.
The next step is the estimation of motion between these gated reconstructions.
This step is crucial as its accuracy highly influences the quality of the final motion
corrected image.

In this chapter we discuss different algorithmic paradigms in terms of *image
registration* and *optical flow* for motion estimation. For both paradigms, a focus is
laid on the preservation of radioactivity (mass-preservation) to incorporate a priori
information. For image registration, different data terms are introduced which are
suitable for monomodal PET registration in combination with mass-preservation.
In particular, a data term adopted to noisy PET data is proposed with the SAD
measure. The preservation of mass requires diffeomorphic transformations to be
a valid assumption. Thus, different regularization schemes will be introduced and
discussed. In addition to the non-parametric transformation model we also present
motion estimation using the popular parametric transformation model based on B-
splines for image registration. For optical flow, classical local and global approaches
are introduced and advanced methods are briefly discussed. In particular, mass-
preserving optical flow in combination with non-quadratic penalization is addressed.
The last part of this chapter compares the two algorithmic paradigms and intends to
provide some guidance to finding an appropriate method for motion estimation and
its configuration in practice.

© The Author(s) 2015
F. Gigengack et al., *Motion Correction in Thoracic Positron Emission Tomography*,
SpringerBriefs in Electrical and Computer Engineering,
DOI 10.1007/978-3-319-08392-6__2

2.1 Image Registration

Image registration is a versatile approach to motion estimation and provides a full range of application-specific options. We give an introduction to image registration including suitable options for the data term in Sect. 2.1.1 and the regularization functional in Sect. 2.1.2. The alternative to non-parametric image registration in terms of B-spline transformations is discussed in Sect. 2.1.3. One of the main messages of this book is the mass-preserving transformation model introduced in Sect. 2.1.4 which is tailored for gated PET. We refer to the comprehensive reviews of image registration for further reading [18, 49, 63, 66, 88, 90, 94, 95, 139].

The aim of image registration is to spatially align two corresponding images. In order to formulate this definition of image registration mathematically, we need to find a way to measure the similarity of two images. The objective is then to find a meaningful spatial transformation that, applied to one of the images, maximizes the similarity.

For motion estimation, a so-called *template image* $\mathcal{T} : \Omega \to \mathbb{R}$ is registered onto a *reference image* $\mathcal{R} : \Omega \to \mathbb{R}$, where $\Omega \subset \mathbb{R}^3$ is the *image domain*. This yields a *spatial transformation* $\mathbf{y} : \mathbb{R}^3 \to \mathbb{R}^3$ representing point-to-point correspondences between $\mathcal{T}$ and $\mathcal{R}$. To find $\mathbf{y}$, the following functional has to be minimized

$$\arg\min_{\mathbf{y}} \; \mathcal{J}(\mathbf{y}) := \mathcal{D}(\mathcal{M}(\mathcal{T}, \mathbf{y}), \, \mathcal{R}) + \alpha \, \mathcal{S}(\mathbf{y}) \, . \tag{2.1}$$

Here $\mathcal{D}$ denotes the *distance functional* measuring the dissimilarity between the transformed template image and the fixed reference image. $\mathcal{M}$ is the *transformation model* specifying how the transformation $\mathbf{y}$ should be applied to the template image $\mathcal{T}$. $\mathcal{S}$ is the *regularization functional* which penalizes non-smooth transformations and thus enforces meaningful solutions.

The standard transformation model is simply given by an interpolation of $\mathcal{T}$ at the transformed grid $\mathbf{y}$

$$\mathcal{M}^{\mathrm{std}}(\mathcal{T}, \mathbf{y}) := \mathcal{T} \circ \mathbf{y} = \mathcal{T}(\mathbf{y}) \, . \tag{2.2}$$

We will discuss an alternative transformation model for mass-preserving image registration in Definition 2.11. A discussion of different options for the data term $\mathcal{D}$ is given in the next Sect. 2.1.1 and for the regularization term $\mathcal{S}$ in Sect. 2.1.2.

2.1.1 Data Terms

The *data term* measures the dissimilarity, i.e., reversal of the similarity, of two input images. In Eq. (2.1) the transformed template image is compared to the reference image. For simplicity we will use the original template image (without transformation) for the following definitions without loss of generality.

(Dis)similarity measures for monomodal registration tasks are best suited for motion correction of gated PET data. We thus restrict the discussion in the rest of this section to these monomodal measures. For a more detailed discussion of similarity measures for multimodal studies, such as mutual information (which measures the amount of shared information of two images) or normalized gradient fields (which measures deviations in the gradients of the input images), we refer to [95].

A common dissimilarity measure for monomodal image registration is SSD, which is introduced in the following Definition. Differences of the reference and the template image are measured quadratically.

Definition 2.1 ($\mathcal{D}^{\mathrm{SSD}}$ – Sum of squared differences). The *sum of squared differences (SSD)* of two images $\mathcal{T} : \Omega \to \mathbb{R}$ and $\mathcal{R} : \Omega \to \mathbb{R}$ on a domain $\Omega \subset \mathbb{R}^3$ is defined as

$$\mathcal{D}^{\mathrm{SSD}}(\mathcal{T}, \mathcal{R}) := \frac{1}{2} \int_{\Omega} (\mathcal{T}(x) - \mathcal{R}(x))^2 \, dx \,. \tag{2.3}$$

SSD measures the point-wise distances of image intensities. For images with locally similar intensities the measure gets low. SSD has to be minimized and has its optimal value at 0.

Large differences in the input images are often induced by noise which consequently leads to a high energy in the data term. L_1-like distance measures are often used in optical flow techniques [19] to overcome this problem. The L_1 distance of two images $\mathcal{T}$ and $\mathcal{R}$ is defined as

$$L_1(\mathcal{T}, \mathcal{R}) := \int_{\Omega} |\mathcal{T}(x) - \mathcal{R}(x)| \, dx \,. \tag{2.4}$$

Using this functional as a data term in Eq. (2.1) raises problems as we require differentiability of all components during optimization. As the absolute value function is not differentiable at zero, the idea is thus to create a differentiable version of the L_1 distance by adding a differentiable outer function ψ to the difference in Eq. (2.4) with a similar behavior to the absolute value function.

Definition 2.2 ($\mathcal{D}^{\mathrm{SAD}}$ – Sum of absolute differences). The (approximated) *sum of absolute differences (SAD)* of two images $\mathcal{T} : \Omega \to \mathbb{R}$ and $\mathcal{R} : \Omega \to \mathbb{R}$ on a domain $\Omega \subset \mathbb{R}^3$ is defined as

$$\mathcal{D}^{\mathrm{SAD}}(\mathcal{T}, \mathcal{R}) := \int_{\Omega} \psi(\mathcal{T}(x) - \mathcal{R}(x)) \, dx \,, \tag{2.5}$$

(continued)

Definition 2.2 (continued)
where $\psi : \mathbb{R} \to \mathbb{R}$ is the continuously differentiable Charbonnier penalizing
function [28] with a small positive constant $\beta \in \mathbb{R}^{>0}$

$$\psi(x) = \sqrt{x^2 + \beta^2} . \qquad (2.6)$$

Remark 2.1. Different choices for the function ψ in Definition 2.2 are possible,
cf. [19].

Remark 2.2. The function ψ in Eq. (2.6) is always greater than zero. Consequently,
$\mathcal{D}^{\mathrm{SAD}}(\mathcal{T}, \mathcal{T}) \neq 0$. This issue could be fixed by subtracting β

$$\hat{\psi}(x) := \sqrt{x^2 + \beta^2} - \beta . \qquad (2.7)$$

For minimization of the registration functional we need to compute the derivatives of the functional and hence the first

$$\partial \psi(x) = \frac{x}{\sqrt{x^2 + \beta^2}} \qquad (2.8)$$

and second derivative of ψ

$$\partial^2 \psi(x) = \frac{\beta^2}{(x^2 + \beta^2)^{3/2}} \qquad (2.9)$$

are given here for completeness.
  The behavior of the penalizing function ψ for different values of β is shown in
Fig. 2.1. It can be observed that ψ becomes more quadratic around zero for higher
β values. This might prevent abrupt jumps in the first derivative between -1 and 1
during optimization, thus stabilizing the optimization process.

2.1.2   Regularization

According to Hadamard [61] a problem is called *well-posed* if there

1. *Exists* a solution that is
2. *Unique* and when
3. Small changes in data lead only to small changes in the result.

In image registration, small changes in the data can lead to large changes in the
results. Further, as the uniqueness is generally not given, image registration is
ill-posed [48]. This makes regularization inevitable and essential to find feasible
transformations.

Regularization restricts the space of possible transformations to a smaller set of reasonable functions. Regularization should be chosen depending on the application and can either be implicit or explicit. If the transformation is regularized by the properties of the space itself, as in parametric image registration, we speak of *implicit regularization*. For example, for a rigid 3D transformation only a total of three rotation and three translation parameters need to be estimated instead of a 3D motion vector for each voxel. In *explicit regularization*, a penalty is added to the registration functional to avoid non-smooth transformations. The penalty is often based on a model that is physically sound and fits the processed data.

As the regularization for parametric transformations is implicitly given we will only analyze penalties for non-linear image registration in this section. In the rest of this section we will introduce the following regularizers:

- Diffusion regularization (Sect. 2.1.2.1),
- Elastic regularization (Sect. 2.1.2.2), and
- Hyperelastic regularization (Sect. 2.1.2.3).

These regularizers are specifically chosen as diffusion regularization is typically used for optical flow applications. Further, VAMPIRE relies on hyperelastic regularization, which is a non-linear generalization of linear elastic regularization. More information about regularization (e.g., curvature or log-elasticity) and additional constraints, which are beyond the scope of this book, can be found in [3, 48, 94, 99, 107].

Hereinafter, we assume a given transformation $y : \mathbb{R}^3 \to \mathbb{R}^3$ which is composed of the spatial position $x \in \mathbb{R}^3$ and a deformation (or displacement) $u : \mathbb{R}^3 \to \mathbb{R}^3$ at position x, i.e., $y(x) = x + u(x)$.

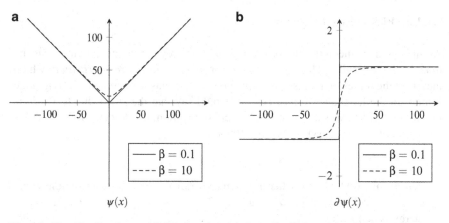

Fig. 2.1 The Charbonnier penalizing function (**a**) from Eq. (2.6) and its derivative (**b**) from Eq. (2.8) are plotted for $\beta = 0.1$ and $\beta = 10$. They both give an approximation to the absolute value function

2.1.2.1 Diffusion Regularization

One of the simplest ways to control the behavior of the transformation is *diffusion regularization* [47]. The basic idea is to disallow large variations in the gradient of the motion vector between neighboring voxels, i.e., oscillations in the deformation u are penalized.

The motivation is thus simply a demanded smoothness of the transformation and no physical one. An advantage of diffusion regularization over other methods is its low computational complexity which allows fast computations and the treatment of high-dimensional data [94]. This becomes important when striving for real-time computations, which is why diffusion regularization is popular for optical flow techniques, cf. Sect. 2.2.

Definition 2.3 ($\mathcal{S}^{\text{diff}}$ – **Diffusion regularization**). For a transformation $y : \mathbb{R}^3 \to \mathbb{R}^3$ with $y(x) = x + u(x)$ and $u : \mathbb{R}^3 \to \mathbb{R}^3$, the *diffusion regularization* energy is defined as

$$\mathcal{S}^{\text{diff}}(u) := \int_{\Omega} \|\nabla u(x)\|_2^2 \, dx = \int_{\Omega} \sum_{i=1}^{3} |\nabla u^i(x)|^2 \, dx , \qquad (2.10)$$

where the (squared) Frobenius norm is defined as $\|A\|_2^2 := \text{tr}(A^T A)$ for matrices $A \in \mathbb{R}^{3 \times 3}$. u^i denotes the i-th component of u with $i \in \{1, 2, 3\}$.

2.1.2.2 Elastic Regularization

As indicated in the introduction of this section, regularization methods can be motivated physically. This is the case for *linear elastic regularization* which measures the forces of a transformation applied to an elastic material [17] (Lagrange frame). In the language of elasticity we would say that the *stress* due to *strain* is measured. Or vice versa, in a more physical motivation, the deformation (*strain*) is a reaction of force (*stress*) [94] (Euler frame).

Definition 2.4 ($\mathcal{S}^{\text{elastic}}$ – **Elastic regularization**). For a transformation $y : \mathbb{R}^3 \to \mathbb{R}^3$ with $y(x) = x + u(x)$ and $u : \mathbb{R}^3 \to \mathbb{R}^3$, the *elastic regularization* energy is defined as

---

(continued)

Definition 2.4 (continued)

$$\mathcal{S}^{\text{elastic}}(\boldsymbol{u}) := \int_{\Omega} \mu \|\nabla \boldsymbol{u}(\boldsymbol{x})\|_2^2 + (\lambda + \mu)(\nabla \cdot \boldsymbol{u}(\boldsymbol{x}))^2 \, d\boldsymbol{x}$$

$$= \int_{\Omega} \mu \left(\sum_{i=1}^{3} |\nabla \boldsymbol{u}^i(\boldsymbol{x})|^2 \right) + (\lambda + \mu) \left(\sum_{i=1}^{3} \boldsymbol{u}_i^i(\boldsymbol{x}) \right)^2 \, d\boldsymbol{x}, (2.11)$$

where $\mu \in \mathbb{R}^{>0}$ and $\lambda \in \mathbb{R}^{>0}$ are the Lamé constants according to Ciarlet [30]. Again, $\|\cdot\|_2$ is the Frobenius norm (see Eq. (2.10)) and $\boldsymbol{u}^i$ denotes the i-th component of $\boldsymbol{u}$ with $i \in \{1, 2, 3\}$.

To better understand the physical interpretation of the elastic energy we will take a look at some useful properties of elasticity in terms of the *Poisson ratio* and *Young's modulus*.

Definition 2.5 (v – **Poisson ratio**). The *Poisson (contraction) ratio* is defined as

$$v = \frac{\lambda}{2(\lambda + \mu)}, \tag{2.12}$$

for the Lamé constants $\mu \in \mathbb{R}^{>0}$ and $\lambda \in \mathbb{R}^{>0}$ in Definition 2.4.

The Poisson ratio v measures the amount of compression for the linear elastic model. If a material is compressed in one direction, the Poisson ratio measures the quotient of this value and the expansion in the other directions. For compressible materials we thus have a small quotient and for incompressible materials a large one. To model incompressible materials in the registration setting, the Poisson ratio needs to be weighted high. Note that this interpretation only holds for small displacements since we are dealing with a linear model.

Definition 2.6 (E – **Young's modulus**). *Young's modulus* is defined as

$$E = \frac{\mu(3\lambda + 2\mu)}{\lambda + \mu}, \tag{2.13}$$

for the Lamé constants $\mu \in \mathbb{R}^{>0}$ and $\lambda \in \mathbb{R}^{>0}$ in Definition 2.4.

Young's modulus E is the quotient of stress (tension) and strain (stretch) in the same direction. The connection between the Lamé constants, Poisson ratio, and Young's modulus is given by

$$\lambda = \frac{Ev}{(1+v)(1-2v)}, \tag{2.14}$$

$$\mu = \frac{E}{2(1+v)}, \tag{2.15}$$

$$\lambda > 0 \text{ and } \mu > 0 \iff 0 < v < \frac{1}{2} \text{ and } E > 0. \tag{2.16}$$

The linear dependency of Young's modulus E and the Lamé constants can be seen in Eqs. (2.14) and (2.15). Together with Eq. (2.11) it gets obvious that E simply scales the regularization functional. For practical reasons it can thus be set to $E = 1$ [73].

2.1.2.3 Hyperelastic Regularization

In many medical applications of image registration the user has a priori knowledge about the processed data concerning the allowed deformations. For example the invertibility of the transformation is a general requirement. More specific knowledge, like, e.g., the degree of compressibility of tissue can also be controlled. We have seen in the linear elastic case that the Poisson ratio (Definition 2.6) gives a measure for compressibility of small deformations. In the non-linear case, the determinant of the Jacobian of the transformation measures the volume change and can thus be used to control the compression behavior – even for large deformations. This is done with polyconvex *hyperelastic regularization* [22, 30, 40]. The regularization functional $\mathcal{S}^{\mathrm{hyper}}$ controls changes in length, area of the surface, and volume of y and guarantees thereby in particular the invertibility of the estimated transformation.

Definition 2.7 ($\mathcal{S}^{\mathrm{hyper}}$ – Hyperelastic regularization). Let $\alpha_l, \alpha_a, \alpha_v \in \mathbb{R}^{>0}$ be constants and $p, q \geq 2$. Further, let $\Gamma_a, \Gamma_v : \mathbb{R} \to \mathbb{R}$ be positive and strictly convex functions, with Γ_v satisfying $\lim_{z \to 0^+} \Gamma_v(z) = \lim_{z \to \infty} \Gamma_v(z) = \infty$. The *hyperelastic regularization* energy caused by the transformation $y : \mathbb{R}^3 \to \mathbb{R}^3$ with $y(x) = x + u(x)$ and $u : \mathbb{R}^3 \to \mathbb{R}^3$ is defined as

$$\mathcal{S}^{\mathrm{hyper}}(y) = \alpha_l \cdot \mathcal{S}^{\mathrm{length}}(y) + \alpha_a \cdot \mathcal{S}^{\mathrm{area}}(y) + \alpha_v \cdot \mathcal{S}^{\mathrm{vol}}(y). \tag{2.17}$$

The three summands individually control changes in length, area of the surface, and volume

$$\mathcal{S}^{\mathrm{length}}(y) := \int_\Omega \|\nabla(y(x) - x)\|_2^p \, dx = \int_\Omega \|\nabla u(x)\|_2^p \, dx \tag{2.18}$$

$$\mathcal{S}^{\mathrm{area}}(y) := \int_\Omega \Gamma_a(\|\mathrm{Cof}(\nabla y(x))\|_2^q) \, dx \tag{2.19}$$

(continued)

Definition 2.7 (continued)

$$\mathcal{S}^{\text{vol}}(\boldsymbol{y}) := \int_{\Omega} \Gamma_v(\det(\nabla \boldsymbol{y}(\boldsymbol{x}))) \, d\boldsymbol{x} \,, \tag{2.20}$$

where $\|\cdot\|_2$ is the Frobenius norm (see Eq. (2.10)) and $\text{Cof}(\cdot)$ denotes the cofactor matrix.

Remark 2.3. A typical choice of p and q in Definition 2.7 is $p = q = 2$ [51].

In the formulation in Eq. (2.1), the positive real number α balances between minimizing the data driven energy term (maximizing the image similarity) and retaining smooth and realistic transformations, which is controlled by the regularization energy. As each term of the hyperelastic regularizer has an individual weighting factor, α can be set to 1 and only α_l, α_a, and α_v need to be determined.

For $\alpha_v > 0$, the conditions for Γ_v claimed above ensure $\det(\nabla \boldsymbol{y}) > 0$, i.e., $\boldsymbol{y}$ is a diffeomorphism [40]. This allows us to omit the absolute value bars later in Eq. (2.45) of the mass-preserving transformation model. Hyperelastic regularization has the ability of modeling tissue characteristics like compressibility, improves the robustness against noise and thus enforces realistic cardiac and respiratory motion estimates.

2.1.2.4 Relations

To deepen the understanding of the regularization energies described in this section, we highlight some similarities and differences. This helps us to understand the relations between the different regularization variants. As we will see in Sect. 2.1.4, controlling volume changes plays an important role in connection with the mass-preserving motion estimation approach VAMPIRE. Accordingly, this aspect is highlighted in particular.

Diffusion $\leftrightarrow$ Elastic

As we have seen, the elastic energy consists of the two terms $\|\nabla \boldsymbol{u}\|_2^2$ and $(\nabla \cdot \boldsymbol{u})^2$. The interpretation of the latter is revealed as a measure of compressibility, i.e., of volume changes. The first term is the known diffusion regularization term, which is hence integrated into the elastic energy.

Diffusion $\leftrightarrow$ Hyperelastic

Diffusion regularization is included into hyperelastic regularization. The length term S^{length} in Eq. 2.17 equals the diffusion regularization term. The hyperelastic regularization energy has two additional energy terms – S^{area} measuring changes in area and S^{vol} measuring changes in volume.

Elastic $\leftrightarrow$ Hyperelastic

The Jacobian determinant $\det(\nabla \mathbf{y})$ represents the exact volume change due to a transformation $\mathbf{y}$. Consequently, a value of one characterizes incompressibility. Let us recall, the Poisson ratio v in the linear elastic model (Definition 2.5) also controls the amount of incompressibility. Large values of v (incompressible) results from large values of λ. For large values of λ compared to μ, the elastic energy is dominated by $(\nabla \cdot \mathbf{u})^2$. The Jacobian determinant can by approximated by $\nabla \cdot \mathbf{u}$ if the $|\partial_j \mathbf{u}^i|$ are sufficiently small:

$$\det(\nabla \mathbf{y}) \approx 1 + \nabla \cdot \mathbf{u} \,. \tag{2.21}$$

This shows the approximate behavior of linear elastic regularization. To conclude, hyperelastic regularization holds for large deformations whereas linear elastic regularization is restricted to small deformations. Further, the area energy term in hyperelastic regularization, which is missing in elastic regularization, serves as a link between the length and volume term [22].

2.1.3 B-Spline Transformation

So far only non-parametric transformations were discussed. However, in some cases the search space for the desired transformation can be restricted by using a suitable parametric transformation model. As an example, for many brain alignment tasks the transformation can be assumed to be rigid. This can increase the robustness of the registration task. The most prominent parametric transformations are scaling, rigid, affine, and spline-based transformations [95]. For non-linear transformations, as required for PET motion estimation, the parametric B-spline transformation is of particular interest.

In parametric image registration the transformation is given in terms of a parametric function $\mathbf{y}_p : \mathbb{R}^3 \to \mathbb{R}^3$. $\mathbf{y}_p$ is defined by a parameter vector p. The task is to find the parameter set p minimizing the distance between $\mathcal{R}$ and the transformed input image $\mathcal{M}(\mathcal{T}, \mathbf{y}_p)$

$$\mathcal{J}(p) := \mathcal{D}(\mathcal{M}(\mathcal{T}, \mathbf{y}_p), \mathcal{R}) \stackrel{!}{=} \min \,, \tag{2.22}$$

where $\mathcal{D}$ is a data term according to Sect. 2.1.1 and $\mathcal{M}$ is a transformation model according to Eq. (2.2) or (2.46).

Definition 2.8 (Spline transformation). Given a number $n = (n^1, n^2, n^3) \in \mathbb{N}^3$ of spline coefficients and a spline basis function $b : \mathbb{R} \to \mathbb{R}$, the *spline transformation* or *free-form transformation* $\mathbf{y}_p(\mathbf{x}) = (y_p^1(\mathbf{x}), y_p^2(\mathbf{x}), y_p^3(\mathbf{x}))$ for a point $\mathbf{x} = (x, y, z)^T \in \Omega \subset \mathbb{R}^3$ is defined as

$$y_p^1(\mathbf{x}) = x + \sum_{i=1}^{n^1} \sum_{j=1}^{n^2} \sum_{k=1}^{n^3} p_{i,j,k}^1 b_i(x) b_j(y) b_k(z) , \qquad (2.23)$$

$$y_p^2(\mathbf{x}) = y + \sum_{i=1}^{n^1} \sum_{j=1}^{n^2} \sum_{k=1}^{n^3} p_{i,j,k}^2 b_i(x) b_j(y) b_k(z) , \qquad (2.24)$$

$$y_p^3(\mathbf{x}) = z + \sum_{i=1}^{n^1} \sum_{j=1}^{n^2} \sum_{k=1}^{n^3} p_{i,j,k}^3 b_i(x) b_j(y) b_k(z) , \qquad (2.25)$$

where

$$p = \left\{ (p_{i,j,k}^1, p_{i,j,k}^2, p_{i,j,k}^3)^T \in \mathbb{R}^3 \mid \right.$$
$$\left. i \in \{1, \ldots, n^1\}, j \in \{1, \ldots, n^2\}, k \in \{1, \ldots, n^3\} \right\} \qquad (2.26)$$

are the spline coefficients and $b_i(x) = b(x - i)$ for $i \in \{1, \ldots, n^1\}$, $b_j(y) = b(y - j)$ for $j \in \{1, \ldots, n^2\}$, $b_k(z) = b(z - k)$ for $k \in \{1, \ldots, n^3\}$. Note that this notation is only valid for $\Omega = \{(x, y, z)^T \in \mathbb{R}^3 \mid 0 \leq x < n^1 + 1, 0 \leq y < n^2 + 1, 0 \leq z < n^3 + 1\}$.

A possible choice for the basis function $b : \mathbb{R} \to \mathbb{R}$, often called *mother spline* (cf. Fig. 2.2), is

$$b(x) = \begin{cases} (x+2)^3 , & -2 \leq x < -1 , \\ -x^3 - 2(x+1)^3 + 6(x+1) , & -1 \leq x < 0 , \\ x^3 + 2(x-1)^3 - 6(x-1) , & 0 \leq x < 1 , \\ (-x+2)^3 , & 1 \leq x < 2 , \\ 0 , & else . \end{cases} \qquad (2.27)$$

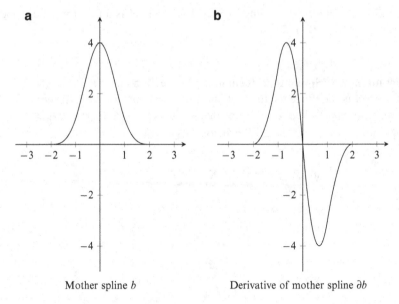

Mother spline b Derivative of mother spline ∂b

Fig. 2.2 The mother spline b defined in Eq. (2.27) is shown in (**a**). b is continuously differentiable and its derivative is plotted in (**b**)

Parametric transformations are implicitly regularized by the reduced number of parameters compared to non-parametric transformations, as discussed in Sect. 2.1.2. Hence, regularization of, e.g., rigid or affine transformations, is usually not necessary. However, regularization becomes of importance for spline transformations due to the non-linearity [48]. Possible regularization variants for spline transformations are discussed in the following. For parametric transformations the functional in Eq. (2.22) becomes

$$\mathcal{J}(p) := \mathcal{D}(\mathcal{M}(\mathcal{T}, \mathbf{y}_p), \mathcal{R}) + \alpha \cdot \mathcal{S}_M(p) \overset{!}{=} \min , \qquad (2.28)$$

for a regularization term $\mathcal{S}_M$ and a scalar weighting factor $\alpha \in \mathbb{R}^{>0}$ balancing between the data and regularization term.

2.1.3.1 Hyperelastic Regularization

Hyperelastic regularization, introduced for non-parametric transformations in Definition 2.7, can also be applied to the B-spline transformation model. The transformation $\mathbf{y}_p(\mathbf{x}) = \mathbf{x} + \mathbf{u}_p(\mathbf{x})$ is written in the discrete setting of [95] as

$$\mathbf{y} = \mathbf{x} + Q \cdot p . \qquad (2.29)$$

The deformation $\boldsymbol{u}$ is represented by a projection of the spline coefficients, given by the parameter vector p, into the image space by the projection matrix Q

$$\boldsymbol{u} = Q \cdot p. \tag{2.30}$$

For the hyperelastic regularization the transformation $\boldsymbol{y}$ is first determined according to Eq. (2.29) and is then regularized as described in Eq. (2.17). The regularization functional in Eq. (2.28) is then defined as

$$\mathcal{S}_M(p) := \mathcal{S}^{\text{hyper}}(\boldsymbol{x} + Q \cdot p). \tag{2.31}$$

2.1.3.2 Coefficient-Based Regularization

The regularization term $\mathcal{S}_M(p)$ in Eq. (2.28) is based on the coefficient vector p in the case of coefficient-based regularization and is a weighted norm of the form

$$\mathcal{S}_M(p) := \|p\|_M^2 := p^T M p. \tag{2.32}$$

The matrix M determines the regularization type. Instead of regularizing the deformation $\boldsymbol{u}_p(\boldsymbol{x})$ for each spatial position $\boldsymbol{x} \in \mathbb{R}^3$ as in the non-parametric case (cf. Sect. 2.1.2) we now regularize directly on p. We speak of coefficient-based regularization in *image space* if the regularization on p considers the projection matrix Q and thus regularizes $Q \cdot p$. If only p is taken into account we speak of coefficient-based regularization in *coefficient space*.

With Tikhonov regularization we will discuss one option for coefficient-based regularization in coefficient space. Tikhonov regularization punishes gradients in the spline coefficients and is the coefficient-based analog of diffusion regularization introduced in Definition 2.3.

Definition 2.9 (Tikhonov regularization (coefficient space)). *Tikhonov regularization* in coefficient space is defined by the choice of

$$M^{\text{tc}} = D^T D \tag{2.33}$$

in Eq. (2.32). The superscript tc denotes (t)ikhonov in (c)oefficient space. D is defined by

$$D = I_3 \otimes \begin{bmatrix} D^1 \\ D^2 \\ D^3 \end{bmatrix}. \tag{2.34}$$

(continued)

Definition 2.9 (continued)
Here I_3 is the 3×3 identity matrix and $\otimes$ denotes the Kronecker product [16]. The 1D derivative operators are defined by

$$D^1 = I_{n^3} \otimes I_{n^2} \otimes d_1^1 \,, \tag{2.35}$$

$$D^2 = I_{n^3} \otimes d_1^2 \otimes I_{n^1} \,, \tag{2.36}$$

$$D^3 = d_1^3 \otimes I_{n^2} \otimes I_{n^1} \,. \tag{2.37}$$

The I_{n^i} denote identity matrices with the size $n^i \times n^i, i \in \{1,2,3\}$, and the n^i defined according to Definition 2.8. The discrete 1D first derivative operators for each dimension are defined by

$$d_1^i = \begin{bmatrix} -1 & 1 & & 0 \\ & \ddots & \ddots & \\ 0 & & -1 & 1 \end{bmatrix} \in \mathbb{R}^{n^i-1,n^i}, \ i \in \{1,2,3\} \,. \tag{2.38}$$

The analog of the above definition in image space is given with the following Definition 2.10. As the real displacements and not the corresponding coefficients are processed, this version is even more related to the diffusion regularization energy in Definition 2.3.

Definition 2.10 (Tikhonov regularization (image space)). Let the number of spline coefficients be $n = (n^1, n^2, n^3) \in \mathbb{N}^3$ and $b_i(x) = b(x - i)$ for $i \in \{1, \ldots, n^d\}$, $d \in \{1, 2, 3\}$, be the translated spline basis function b defined in Eq. (2.27). The *Tikhonov regularization* matrix in image space is defined as

$$M^{\text{ti}} = I_3 \otimes T^3 \otimes T^2 \otimes T^1 \,. \tag{2.39}$$

The matrices $T^d \in \mathbb{R}^{n^d, n^d}$ are defined by

$$T_{i,j}^d = \int_{\Omega^d} \partial b_i(x) \cdot \partial b_j(x) dx \,, \ d \in \{1, 2, 3\} \,, \tag{2.40}$$

where $i \in \{1, \ldots, n^d\}$, $j \in \{1, \ldots, n^d\}$, and $\Omega^d \subset \mathbb{R}$ is the 1D subspace of Ω in dimension $d \in \{1, 2, 3\}$.

(continued)

Definition 2.10 (continued)

The concrete numbers for the matrix T^d (including boundary treatment) are

$$T^d = \begin{bmatrix} 15.1 & -5.0 & -7.2 & -0.3 & & & & & & 0 \\ -5.0 & 23.9 & -4.5 & -7.2 & -0.3 & & & & & \\ -7.2 & -4.5 & 24.0 & -4.5 & -7.2 & -0.3 & & & & \\ -0.3 & -7.2 & -4.5 & 24.0 & -4.5 & -7.2 & -0.3 & & & \\ & \ddots & \ddots & \ddots & \ddots & \ddots & \ddots & \ddots & & \\ & & -0.3 & -7.2 & -4.5 & 24.0 & -4.5 & -7.2 & -0.3 & \\ & & & -0.3 & -7.2 & -4.5 & 24.0 & -4.5 & -7.2 & \\ & & & & -0.3 & -7.2 & -4.5 & 23.9 & -5.0 & \\ 0 & & & & & -0.3 & -7.2 & -5.0 & 15.1 \end{bmatrix} \in \mathbb{R}^{n^d, n^d}$$

$$(2.41)$$

for $d \in \{1,2,3\}$. The entries of the matrix T^d are obtained by calculating the integral in Eq. (2.40) for each index $i \in \{1,\dots,n^d\}$ and $j \in \{1,\dots,n^d\}$, $d \in \{1,2,3\}$.

2.1.4 Mass-Preserving Image Registration

The standard transformation model for image registration in Eq. (2.2) does not guarantee the preservation of mass, i.e., in general

$$\int_\Omega \mathcal{T}(\boldsymbol{x}) \, d\boldsymbol{x} \neq \int_\Omega \mathcal{T}(\boldsymbol{y}(\boldsymbol{x})) \, d\boldsymbol{x} . \qquad (2.42)$$

Further, the distance functional $\mathcal{D}$ typically entails the assumption of similar intensities at corresponding points. This assumption is not valid for the standard transformation model $\mathcal{M}^{\mathrm{std}}$ in case of dual gated PET as discussed in connection with Fig. 1.11. Consequently, the standard transformation model needs some modification to express this feature.

The requirement for the desired transformation model $\mathcal{M}^{\mathrm{MP}}$ is the preservation of mass

$$\int_\Omega \mathcal{T}(\boldsymbol{x}) d\boldsymbol{x} = \int_\Omega \mathcal{M}^{\mathrm{MP}}(\mathcal{T}, \boldsymbol{y}(\boldsymbol{x})) \, d\boldsymbol{x} . \qquad (2.43)$$

From the integration by substitution theorem for multiple variables we know that the following equation holds

$$\int_{y(\Omega)} T(x)\, dx = \int_{\Omega} T(y(x))\, |\det(\nabla y(x))|\, dx \,. \tag{2.44}$$

With respect to PET, Eq. (2.44) guarantees already the same total amount of radioactivity before and after applying the transformation y to T. The Jacobian determinant $|\det(\nabla y(x))|$ accounts for the volume change induced by the transformation y, representing the mass-preserving component. As y should reflect cardiac and respiratory motion, transformations that are not bijective are anatomically not meaningful and have therefore to be excluded. For example, the hyperelastic regularization functional in Sect. 2.1.2.3 guarantees y to be diffeomorphic and orientation preserving, which allows us to drop the absolute value bars

$$\int_{y(\Omega)} T(x)dx = \int_{\Omega} T(y(x))\, \det(\nabla y(x))\, dx \,. \tag{2.45}$$

We derived the VAMPIRE (Variational Algorithm for Mass-Preserving Image REgistration) based on the above considerations in our previous work [51]. The source code of VAMPIRE can be downloaded at [52].

Definition 2.11 ($\mathcal{M}^{MP}$ – Mass-preserving transformation model). For an image $T : \Omega \to \mathbb{R}$ on the domain $\Omega \subset \mathbb{R}^3$ and a transformation $y : \mathbb{R}^3 \to \mathbb{R}^3$ the *mass-preserving transformation model* is defined as

$$\mathcal{M}^{MP}(T, y) := (T \circ y) \cdot \det(\nabla y) = T(y) \cdot \det(\nabla y) \,. \tag{2.46}$$

In the mass-preserving transformation model of VAMPIRE the template image T is transformed by interpolation on the deformed grid y with an additional multiplication by the volume change. The multiplication by the Jacobian is a physiological and realistic modeling for density-based images [128, 138]. It guarantees similar intensities at corresponding points after transformation with a simultaneous preservation of the total amount of radioactivity.

A simple 2D example for the mass-preserving transformation model is shown in Fig. 2.3 for illustration. We will use the same notation as in the 3D case for T, R, Ω, y, and x. Thus, we redefine $\Omega \subset \mathbb{R}^2$, $y : \mathbb{R}^2 \to \mathbb{R}^2$, and $x = (x, y)^T \in \mathbb{R}^2$ for the 2D example. $T : \Omega \to \mathbb{R}$ and $R : \Omega \to \mathbb{R}$ are defined in the same way but for the new domain Ω.

The images of the example are constructed to be similar to SA views of the heart to a certain degree, cf. Fig. 1.14b. Further, they have the same total mass (by construction) and thus exactly fulfill the conditions for mass-preservation. The template and reference image represent smooth signals based on Gaussian distributions. The template image is created by subtracting two Gaussian distributions with different standard deviation $\sigma_1, \sigma_2 \in \mathbb{R}^{>0}$ and $\sigma_1 > \sigma_2$

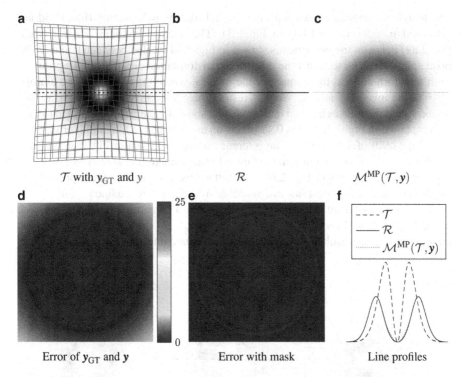

Fig. 2.3 2D example for the mass-preserving transformation model. The template image $\mathcal{T}$ in (**a**) is registered to the reference image $\mathcal{R}$ in (**b**) with VAMPIRE resulting in (**c**). The average endpoint error e between the estimated transformation $\mathbf{y}$ and the ground-truth transformation $\mathbf{y}_{\text{GT}}$ is visualized in (**d**). The same plot restricted to a mask where $\mathcal{T}$ and $\mathcal{R}$ have an intensity above 1 is shown in (**e**). The color map for both error plots is given in-between. Line profiles are shown in (**f**). (Colored figures are only available in the online version.)

$$\mathcal{T}(\mathbf{x}) := g(\mathbf{x}, \sigma_1) - g(\mathbf{x}, \sigma_2) , \tag{2.47}$$

with

$$g(\mathbf{x}, \sigma) := \frac{1}{2\pi\sigma^2} \cdot e^{-\frac{x^2 + y^2}{2\sigma^2}} . \tag{2.48}$$

The intensities are finally scaled between 0 and 255. The reference image $\mathcal{R}$ is created by applying a known transformation $\mathbf{y}_{\text{GT}}$ to $\mathcal{T}$ according to the mass-preserving transformation model $\mathcal{M}^{\text{MP}}(\mathcal{T}, \mathbf{y}_{\text{GT}})$ in Eq. (2.46). Hence, $\mathcal{T}$ and $\mathcal{R}$ have the same global mass. The ground-truth transformation is defined by

$$\mathbf{y}_{\text{GT}}(\mathbf{x}) := \begin{pmatrix} x \cdot (1 - \frac{1}{2} g(\mathbf{x}, \sigma_3)) \\ y \cdot (1 - \frac{1}{2} g(\mathbf{x}, \sigma_3)) \end{pmatrix} , \quad \sigma_3 \in \mathbb{R}^{>0} . \tag{2.49}$$

The template image is shown with the ground-truth transformation (blue) and an estimated transformation (red) in Fig. 2.3a. The average endpoint error e from Eq. (2.89) between the two grids is shown in Fig. 2.3d (scaled between 0 and 25 in pixel units). It can be seen that the estimated transformation differs from the ground-truth transformation at the corners of the images, where the intensities are almost zeros in the images $\mathcal{T}$ and $\mathcal{R}$. We thus restrict the quantitative error analysis to the region where the images have an intensity value above 1. The error e restricted to this area is shown in Fig. 2.3e and is 0.47 pixels on average with a maximum error $e^{\max}$ from Eq. (2.90) of 1.39 pixels. The reference image is shown in Fig. 2.3b and the resulting image after applying the estimated transformation is shown in Fig. 2.3c. Line profiles are given in Fig. 2.3f. The dotted line profile after mass-preserving motion estimation is almost indistinguishable from the reference line profile.

The same experiment is performed for the standard transformation model defined in Eq. (2.2) and is shown in Fig. 2.4. The estimated grid in Fig. 2.4a is subject to major errors which results in an erroneous transformed image in Fig. 2.4c. The error

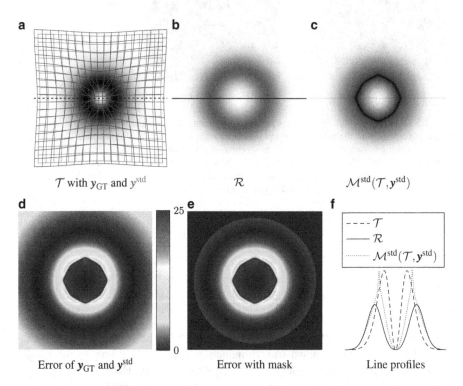

Fig. 2.4 2D example for the standard transformation model. The template image $\mathcal{T}$ in (**a**) is registered to the reference image $\mathcal{R}$ in (**b**) with the standard transformation model in Eq. (2.2) resulting in (**c**). The average endpoint error e between the estimated transformation $\mathbf{y}^{\mathrm{std}}$ and the ground-truth transformation $\mathbf{y}_{\mathrm{GT}}$ is visualized in (**d**). The same plot restricted to a mask where $\mathcal{T}$ and $\mathcal{R}$ have an intensity above 1 is shown in (**e**). The color map for both error plots is given in-between. Line profiles are shown in (**f**). (Colored figures are only available in the online version.)

e (restricted to the same area as discussed above) is shown in Fig. 2.4e (scaled between 0 and 25) and is 4.08 pixels on average with a maximum endpoint error $e^{\max}$ of 17.11 pixels. This simple 2D example thus shows that the mass-preserving motion model is mandatory for density-based images with varying intensities at corresponding points.

2.1.5 Multi-level Optimization

The image registration problem, in terms of minimizing the functional $\mathcal{J}$ in Eq. (2.1), is solved following a discretize-then-optimize approach as in [95]. Discrete objective functionals are obtained by discretizing the objective functional on a coarse to fine hierarchy of levels. On each level the discrete problem can be solved using standard optimization methods, like for instance Gauss-Newton, (l-)BFGS or Trust Region [100]. A short introduction to these methods is given in Sects. 2.1.5.1–2.1.5.3.

It has to be stressed that careful discretization is required to ensure that numerical solutions are meaningful. This is of particular importance for mass-preserving transformations where it is assumed that $\det(\nabla y(x)) > 0$ for all $x \in \Omega$. Discretization of these constraints is known to be extremely challenging and has been discussed in detail in [59, 60]. Using the discretization of the hyperelastic regularization functional derived in [22] we can assure positive Jacobean determinants.

We next discuss the *multi-level* strategy which is similar to cascadic multi-grid [15]. We begin by solving a discrete optimization on a very coarse level which thus has only a small number of unknowns. The coarse transformation is then interpolated to the next finer level and used as a starting guess for the minimization of the next objective function. The procedure is repeated until the transformation is of desired resolution. Typically, the image data is simplified as well. Multiple versions of the original images are constructed by iteratively down-sampling the data by a factor around $\frac{1}{2}$. Thus, for 3D data a voxel on a lower level is, e.g., created by averaging 8 neighboring voxels of the next higher level. Variants like using a Gaussian smoothing during down-sampling are also common. An example for multi-level data is given in Fig. 2.5.

There are several advantages of multi-level schemes. First, the danger of being trapped in a local minimum is reduced as only major image features drive the registration on a coarse level. Second, methods such as Gauss-Newton converge faster for a starting guess close to the minimum. Third, solving the coarse grid problems is computationally dramatically cheaper and in most cases only a small number of correction steps are required on the finer levels. The principle of multi-level image registration is summarized in Algorithm 2.1.

An artificial example for the potential behavior of the objective function is given in Fig. 2.6. The objective function on the lowest level (coarse level) shows a smooth behavior and thus allows a fast and robust initial guess of the global minimum. With increasing resolution level the additional information in the images leads to a less smooth behavior of the function.

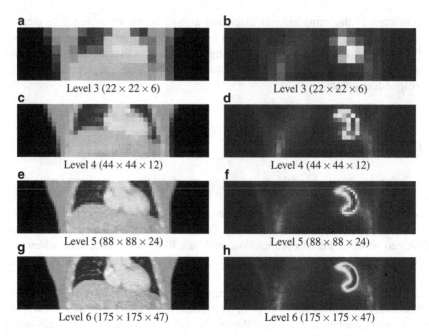

Fig. 2.5 Multi-Level: The central coronal slice in y-direction is shown for different resolution levels. The different levels of a CT scan are shown in the *left column* and corresponding PET images are shown in the *right column*. (**a**) Level 3 ($22 \times 22 \times 6$) (**b**) Level 3 ($22 \times 22 \times 6$) (**c**) Level 4 ($44 \times 44 \times 12$) (**d**) Level 4 ($44 \times 44 \times 12$) (**e**) Level 5 ($88 \times 88 \times 24$) (**f**) Level 5 ($88 \times 88 \times 24$) (**g**) Level 6 ($175 \times 175 \times 47$) (**h**) Level 6 ($175 \times 175 \times 47$)

Algorithm 2.1 Multi-level image registration

Input: Template image $\mathcal{T}$ and reference image $\mathcal{R}$
Output: Transformation $\mathbf{y}$
  $\mathbf{y}_{\text{minLevel}} \leftarrow \mathbf{1}$ // initialize transformation with identity
  for level = minLevel $\rightarrow$ maxLevel **do**
    $\mathcal{T}_{\text{level}} \leftarrow \mathcal{T}$ // down-sampling of template image
    $\mathcal{R}_{\text{level}} \leftarrow \mathcal{R}$ // down-sampling of reference image
    $\mathbf{y}_{\text{level}} \leftarrow \operatorname{argmin} \mathcal{J}(\mathbf{y}_{\text{level}})$ // update motion by minimizing the functional
    if level < maxLevel **then**
      $\mathbf{y}_{\text{level}+1} \leftarrow \mathbf{y}_{\text{level}}$ // prolongate transformation to next level
    end if
  end for
  $\mathbf{y} \leftarrow \mathbf{y}_{\text{maxLevel}}$ // output final transformation

---

We will meet the general multi-level idea again in optical flow motion estimation in Sect. 2.2, as it allows to estimate large deformations with optical flow. However, the approach presented here still differs from the optimize-then-discretize approach that is typically used in optical flow, cf. Sect. 2.2. Most importantly, the discretization used here guarantees that the solution fulfills the properties assumed in the theory on each discretization level and that large steps can be taken in the numerical optimization. Also optimization techniques are well understood and clear rules for stopping [55], step lengths [1, 100], etc. exist.

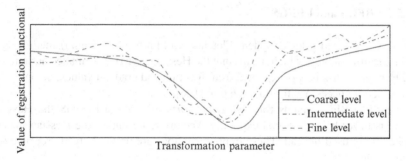

Fig. 2.6 Artificial example for the behavior of an objective function in a multi-level setting. For each level, going from the coarse to the fine level, the value of the registration functional is plotted against the (artificial) transformation parameter. With increasing level, the function is getting less smooth due to the increased level of details in the images. Note the slight shift of the global minimum between the different levels

2.1.5.1 Gauss-Newton

The minimization of the discretized registration functional $\mathcal{J}$ can be solved by means of the Gauss-Newton method. To this end, we can approximate the functional in Eq. (2.1) by a Taylor expansion (leaving the regularization term aside)

$$\mathcal{J}(y + \nabla y) \approx \mathcal{J}(y) + \nabla \mathcal{J}(y) \nabla y + \frac{1}{2}(\nabla y)^T (\nabla^2 \mathcal{J}(x))(\nabla y)$$

$$= \mathcal{J} + \nabla \mathcal{J} \nabla y + \frac{1}{2}(\nabla y)^T H(\nabla y), \qquad (2.50)$$

where H is the (approximated) Hessian matrix. Let us assume the functional $\mathcal{J}$ is given by a residual $r(y)$ and an outer function $\psi(\cdot)$. In the case of SSD this is $r(y) = \mathcal{T} \circ y - \mathcal{R}$ and $\psi(x) = \frac{1}{2}x^2$. The Hessian matrix H is then approximated by

$$H = \nabla^2 \mathcal{J}(x) = \nabla r(x)^T \, \nabla^2 \psi \, \nabla r(x). \qquad (2.51)$$

According to [95] a minimizer of $\mathcal{J}$ is then given by

$$H \nabla y = -\nabla \mathcal{J}. \qquad (2.52)$$

The last step in the Gauss-Newton method is the search for an adequate step size for the motion update ∇y. The updated transformation should reduce the objective function's value compared to the previous guess. A simple way to do this is the Armijo line search. The idea is to add the previously determined search direction to the transformation with decreasing step size (it is halved in each step) until a reduction of the objective function's value occurs.

2.1.5.2 BFGS and l-BFGS

The BFGS (named after Broyden, Fletcher, Goldfarb, and Shanno) method is a quasi-Newton method, which means that the Hessian matrix is estimated at runtime. The Hessian matrix is approximated from function and gradient values. So only first derivatives are necessary for optimization [100].

The l in l-BFGS stands for *limited memory* [85, 95]. In l-BFGS the Hessian matrix is never built or stored explicitly. Vectors representing the Hessian matrix implicitly are used instead. These implementations are particularly appropriate for large problems.

2.1.5.3 Trust Region

In trust region optimization the objective function is treated only in a small (trusted) region where it is approximated by a quadratic model. This is a somehow reverse approach to line search methods. In trust region methods the step size is chosen first (in terms of the region size) and the search direction is computed subsequently. The proceeding in line search methods is vice versa: given a search direction, an appropriate step size is searched.

2.1.6 *Results*

Software phantoms like the XCAT phantom [123] are helpful to validate the proposed motion estimation algorithms as they provide morphological (anatomy) and functional (physiology) ground-truth information. The XCAT phantom is popular in emission tomography for human anatomy as it provides a model of the subject's anatomy and physiology. It is possible to include respiratory and cardiac motion resulting in 4D/5D images. In addition to the generation of PET images and attenuation maps, the XCAT phantom provides information about the ground-truth motion being used to generate the different motion states. This motion information can thus be used to quantitatively evaluate the estimated motion fields of the motion estimation approaches. Some results based on the ground-truth motion are given in Sect. 2.3.

For the evaluation in the following, a 5-by-5 dual gating data set is generated with the XCAT software phantom. The maximum diaphragm motion is set to 20 mm and the dual gates cover the whole range of the breathing and cardiac cycle. The total size of each volume is $175 \times 175 \times 47$ with a voxel size of 3.375 mm in each dimension, simulating the Siemens Biograph^{TM} Sensation 16 PET/CT scanner (Siemens Medical Solution).

The XCAT phantom data is trimmed to be comparable to real patient data in terms of tracer distribution, noise, and the scanning system, cf. [51]. To simulate nearly realistic PET images the following steps are performed:

1. Blurring with a Gaussian kernel (simulation of the PVE),
2. Forward projection,
3. Simulation of Poisson noise, and
4. Reconstruction.

The Gaussian kernel is chosen with a FWHM of 3.85 mm according to the simulated scanner [51]. The blurred images are forward projected into measurement space, where Poisson noise is simulated. The amount of noise is adjusted approximately equal to real patient data. In a final step, the sinograms are reconstructed with the EMRECON software [78]. It should be mentioned that the image acquisition process could alternatively be simulated using the simulation tool *GATE* [69].

We applied the proposed VAMPIRE approach, once with the SSD and once with the SAD distance measure, to the XCAT data. The results of the SSD and SAD VAMPIRE approach are visualized in Figs. 2.7 respectively 2.8 for one representative slice. The gate in maximum inspiration and systole, shown in each case in Fig. 2.7a, is chosen as the template image $\mathcal{T}$, as it is the most different gate compared to the reference image $\mathcal{R}$ in maximum expiration and diastole, shown in Fig. 2.7b. Additionally, the transformed image according to the estimated transformation, i.e., $\mathcal{M}^{MP}(\mathcal{T}, \mathbf{y}_{SSD})$ and $\mathcal{M}^{MP}(\mathcal{T}, \mathbf{y}_{SAD})$, and a vector plot are given in Fig. 2.7c, d. Some quantitative numbers based on the ground-truth transformation are further given at the end of Sect. 2.3 for the VAMPIRE results and the Mass-Preserving Optical Flow (MPOF) approach described in the next section.

2.2 Optical Flow

The motion between two images can not only be estimated by means of image registration. A common alternative is the so-called *optical flow*. The objective is indeed the same, but the problem formulation and implementation are different. Optical flow algorithms are used to estimate a dense flow field between two images/volumes.

In this section we will first derive the basic equation of optical flow. It will directly lead us to the early works on this topic: the local approach of Lucas and Kanade in Sect. 2.2.1 and the global approach of Horn and Schunck in Sect. 2.2.2. Advanced optical flow methods will be discussed in Sect. 2.2.3. A mass-preserving optical flow algorithm will be presented in Sect. 2.2.4. After a brief discussion of a multi-level implementation in Sect. 2.2.5 we finally present some results in Sect. 2.2.6.

The basic idea behind optical flow estimation is that the intensity of a voxel $\mathbf{x}^T = (x, y, z) \in \mathbb{R}^3$ remains constant over time. While changing its spatial position, the intensity of a moving point does not change. This constraint is called *brightness constancy constraint* and can be formulated for 3D volumes as

$$\mathcal{I}(x, y, z, t) = \mathcal{I}(x + u, y + v, z + w, t + 1), \tag{2.53}$$

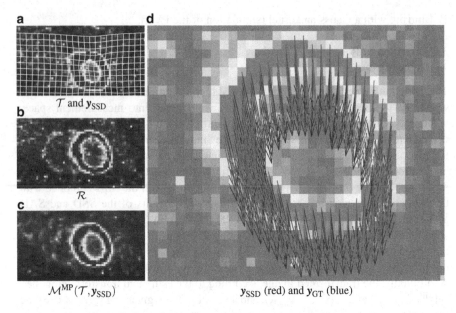

a $\mathcal{T}$ and $\mathbf{y}_{\text{SSD}}$

b $\mathcal{R}$

c $\mathcal{M}^{\text{MP}}(\mathcal{T}, \mathbf{y}_{\text{SSD}})$

d $\mathbf{y}_{\text{SSD}}$ (red) and $\mathbf{y}_{\text{GT}}$ (blue)

Fig. 2.7 SSD VAMPIRE: $\mathcal{T}$ in (**a**) is registered to $\mathcal{R}$ in (**b**) leading to the overlaid transformation grid in (**a**). The transformed template image is shown in (**c**). A magnification with a comparison of the estimated vectors (*red*) and the ground-truth vectors (*blue*) is shown in (**d**). (Colored figures are only available in the online version.)

where $\mathcal{I} : \Omega \times \mathbb{R} \to \mathbb{R}$ denotes the *image* on the *domain* $\Omega \subset \mathbb{R}^3$ and $t \in \mathbb{R}$ the *time*. The *flow* or *displacement* is given by $\boldsymbol{u}^T = (u, v, w, 1) \in \mathbb{R}^4$ for the three spatial dimensions and one time step.

A Taylor linearization in the point $\mathbf{x}$ is applied to $\mathcal{I}(x+u, y+v, z+w, t+1)$ which is valid for small displacements, resulting in

$$\mathcal{I}(x+u, y+v, z+w, t+1) = \mathcal{I}(x, y, z, t)$$

$$+ \frac{\partial}{\partial x}\mathcal{I}(x, y, z, t) \cdot u$$

$$+ \frac{\partial}{\partial y}\mathcal{I}(x, y, z, t) \cdot v \qquad (2.54)$$

$$+ \frac{\partial}{\partial z}\mathcal{I}(x, y, z, t) \cdot w$$

$$+ \frac{\partial}{\partial t}\mathcal{I}(x, y, z, t)$$

$$+ \text{higher order terms.}$$

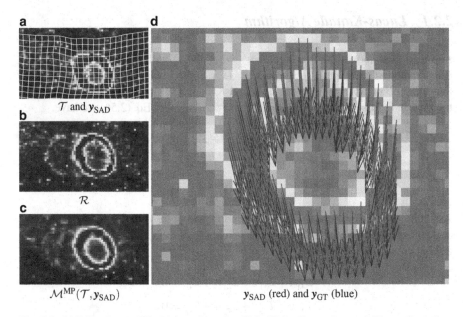

a

$\mathcal{T}$ and $\mathbf{y}_{\text{SAD}}$

b

$\mathcal{R}$

c

$\mathcal{M}^{\text{MP}}(\mathcal{T},\mathbf{y}_{\text{SAD}})$

d

$\mathbf{y}_{\text{SAD}}$ (red) and $\mathbf{y}_{\text{GT}}$ (blue)

Fig. 2.8 SAD VAMPIRE: $\mathcal{T}$ in (**a**) is registered to $\mathcal{R}$ in (**b**) leading to the overlaid transformation grid in (**a**). The transformed template image is shown in (**c**). A magnification with a comparison of the estimated vectors (*red*) and the ground-truth vectors (*blue*) is shown in (**d**). (Colored figures are only available in the online version.)

Inserting Eq. (2.54) into (2.53) leads to

$$
\begin{aligned}
0 &= \frac{\partial}{\partial x}\mathcal{I}(x,y,z,t)\cdot u + \frac{\partial}{\partial y}\mathcal{I}(x,y,z,t)\cdot v + \frac{\partial}{\partial z}\mathcal{I}(x,y,z,t)\cdot w + \frac{\partial}{\partial t}\mathcal{I}(x,y,z,t) \\
&= \mathcal{I}_x u + \mathcal{I}_y v + \mathcal{I}_z w + \mathcal{I}_t \\
&= \mathbf{u}^T \nabla \mathcal{I}\,.
\end{aligned}
$$

$$(2.55)$$

For the sake of notation simplicity we will use the shortterm $\mathcal{I}$ for $\mathcal{I}(\mathbf{x},t)$ in the following. The terms $\mathcal{I}_x$, $\mathcal{I}_y$, and $\mathcal{I}_z$ above represent the derivatives of $\mathcal{I}$. Similarly, $\mathbf{u}(\mathbf{x})$ is shortened to $\mathbf{u}$. Equation (2.55) immediately gives us the data term for standard optical flow algorithms.

$$
\mathbf{D}(\mathcal{I},\mathbf{u})^2 := (\mathbf{u}^T\nabla\mathcal{I})^2 = (\mathcal{I}_x u + \mathcal{I}_y v + \mathcal{I}_z w + \mathcal{I}_t)^2\,.
$$

$$(2.56)$$

As we now have an equation in three variables (the motion along the three directions) additional conditions have to be formulated to make the problem solvable. Different conditions have been proposed to this end.

2.2.1 Lucas-Kanade Algorithm

As mentioned above, the flow vector $u^T = (u, v, w, 1)$ with three unknowns has to be estimated at each spatial position $x^T = (x, y, z)$. To obtain an equation system so that the problem can be solved, Lucas and Kanade [86] made the assumption that the motion field is constant in a small area around x. With Eq. (2.56) we have

$$\mathcal{I}_x u + \mathcal{I}_y v + \mathcal{I}_z w + \mathcal{I}_t = 0 \tag{2.57}$$

or

$$u^T \nabla \mathcal{I} = 0 . \tag{2.58}$$

Assuming a constant flow u in a small window of size $m \times m \times m$, $m > 1$, centered at the voxel position x and denoting the neighbors as (x_i, y_i, z_i), $i = 1, \dots, n$, we get a set of equations

$$
\begin{aligned}
\mathcal{I}_{x_1} u + \mathcal{I}_{y_1} v + \mathcal{I}_{z_1} w + \mathcal{I}_{t_1} &= 0 \\
\mathcal{I}_{x_2} u + \mathcal{I}_{y_2} v + \mathcal{I}_{z_2} w + \mathcal{I}_{t_2} &= 0 \\
\vdots \qquad \vdots \qquad \vdots \qquad \\
\mathcal{I}_{x_n} u + \mathcal{I}_{y_n} v + \mathcal{I}_{z_n} w + \mathcal{I}_{t_n} &= 0
\end{aligned}
\tag{2.59}
$$

where $\mathcal{I}_{x_i}$, $\mathcal{I}_{y_i}$, $\mathcal{I}_{z_i}$, and $\mathcal{I}_{t_i}$, $i = 1, \dots, n$, represent the shortterm for $\mathcal{I}_x(x_i, y_i, z_i, t)$, $\mathcal{I}_y(x_i, y_i, z_i, t)$, $\mathcal{I}_z(x_i, y_i, z_i, t)$, and $\mathcal{I}_t(x_i, y_i, z_i, t)$, respectively. Usually the central voxel is given more weight to suppress noise and thus a Gaussian weighting function is applied to obtain a modified data term [135]

$$\mathbf{D}_{\mathrm{LK}}(\mathcal{I}, u)^2 := u^T (G * (\nabla \mathcal{I} \nabla \mathcal{I}^T)) u , \tag{2.60}$$

where G is a Gaussian smoothing kernel which is convolved component-wisely with the image gradients $\nabla \mathcal{I} \nabla \mathcal{I}^T$ of the neighboring voxels. This minimization problem is solved in a standard least-squares manner.

The optical flow estimated with the Lucas-Kanade algorithm fades out quickly with increasing distance from the motion boundaries. The method is comparatively robust in presence of noise [9, 19].

Algorithm 2.2 Lucas-Kanade optical flow method

Input: Images $\mathcal{I}(x, t)$ and $\mathcal{I}(x, t+1)$
Output: Motion estimate u (for all voxels)
   estimate $\nabla \mathcal{I}$ of each voxel for $\mathcal{I}(x, t)$
  for each voxel x **do**
     compute $u(x)$ by least-squares based minimization of Eq. (2.60)
  end for

2.2.2 Horn-Schunck Algorithm

Another option to make the ill-posed problem solvable is to assume an additional condition of smoothness in flow. This condition is used in the seminal work of Horn and Schunck [64]. Globally smooth motion field means that it varies only little between neighbouring voxels. Thus, they apply a homogeneous diffusion regularization term to the optical flow functional in Eq. (2.56), cf. Sect. 2.1.2.1. In this way a new energy functional consisting of a data term and a smoothness term is built which is to be minimized to get the optical flow

$$\mathcal{J}_{HS}(\boldsymbol{u}) = \int_{\Omega} \mathbf{D}(\mathcal{I}, \boldsymbol{u})^2 d\boldsymbol{x} + \alpha \int_{\Omega} \mathbf{S}(\boldsymbol{u}) d\boldsymbol{x}, \qquad (2.61)$$

where $\mathbf{S}(\boldsymbol{u})$ is the diffusion regularization energy

$$\mathbf{S}(\boldsymbol{u}) = |\nabla u|^2 + |\nabla v|^2 + |\nabla w|^2. \qquad (2.62)$$

The parameter α is a regularization constant. Larger values of α lead to a smoother flow field.

The functional in Eq. (2.61) can be minimized by solving the corresponding Euler-Lagrange equations

$$\Delta u - \frac{1}{\alpha^2} \mathcal{I}_x (\mathcal{I}_x u + \mathcal{I}_y v + \mathcal{I}_z w + \mathcal{I}_t) = 0$$

$$\Delta v - \frac{1}{\alpha^2} \mathcal{I}_y (\mathcal{I}_x u + \mathcal{I}_y v + \mathcal{I}_z w + \mathcal{I}_t) = 0 \qquad (2.63)$$

$$\Delta w - \frac{1}{\alpha^2} \mathcal{I}_z (\mathcal{I}_x u + \mathcal{I}_y v + \mathcal{I}_z w + \mathcal{I}_t) = 0$$

where Δ denotes the Laplace operator

$$\Delta = \frac{\partial^2}{\partial x^2} + \frac{\partial^2}{\partial y^2} + \frac{\partial^2}{\partial z^2}.$$

Using the standard approximation of the Laplace operator in image processing: $\Delta f = \bar{f} - f$, $f = u, v, w$, where $\bar{f}$ is the average of f in the neighborhood of the current voxel position, we arrive at the equation system

$$\begin{pmatrix} \alpha^2 + \mathcal{I}_x^2 & \mathcal{I}_x \mathcal{I}_y & \mathcal{I}_x \mathcal{I}_z \\ \mathcal{I}_x \mathcal{I}_y & \alpha^2 + \mathcal{I}_y^2 & \mathcal{I}_y \mathcal{I}_z \\ \mathcal{I}_x \mathcal{I}_z & \mathcal{I}_y \mathcal{I}_z & \alpha^2 + I_z^2 \end{pmatrix} \begin{pmatrix} u \\ v \\ w \end{pmatrix} = \begin{pmatrix} \alpha^2 \bar{u} - \mathcal{I}_x \mathcal{I}_t \\ \alpha^2 \bar{v} - \mathcal{I}_y \mathcal{I}_t \\ \alpha^2 \bar{w} - \mathcal{I}_z \mathcal{I}_t \end{pmatrix}.$$

Solving this system leads to the following iterative scheme

$$u^{k+1} = \overline{u^k} - I_x \cdot \frac{I_x\overline{u^k} + I_y\overline{v^k} + I_z\overline{w^k} + I_t}{\alpha^2 + I_x^2 + I_y^2 + I_z^2}$$

$$v^{k+1} = \overline{v^k} - I_y \cdot \frac{I_x\overline{u^k} + I_y\overline{v^k} + I_z\overline{w^k} + I_t}{\alpha^2 + I_x^2 + I_y^2 + I_z^2} \qquad (2.64)$$

$$w^{k+1} = \overline{w^k} - I_z \cdot \frac{I_x\overline{u^k} + I_y\overline{v^k} + I_z\overline{w^k} + I_t}{\alpha^2 + I_x^2 + I_y^2 + I_z^2}$$

where the superscript k denotes the iteration number.

An advantage of the Horn-Schunck algorithm is that it yields a high density of flow vectors, i.e., the flow information missing in inner parts of homogeneous objects is *filled in* from the motion boundaries. However, it is more sensitive to noise than local methods [19, 93].

Algorithm 2.3 Horn-Schunck optical flow method

Input: Images $\mathcal{I}(\boldsymbol{x}, t)$ and $\mathcal{I}(\boldsymbol{x}, t+1)$
Output: Motion estimate $\boldsymbol{u}$ (for all voxels)
   compute $\nabla\mathcal{I}$ for each voxel $\boldsymbol{x}$ of $\mathcal{I}(\boldsymbol{x}, t)$
   initialize $\boldsymbol{u}$ for all voxels, e.g., null vector
   while change in $\boldsymbol{u} >$ threshold **do**
      for each voxel $\boldsymbol{x}$ **do**
         compute $\boldsymbol{u}(\boldsymbol{x})$ as given in Eqs. (2.64)
      end for
   end while

2.2.3   Advanced Optical Flow Algorithms

In the literature exists a substantial amount of recent work that improve the basic local and global optical flow approaches in various ways. As stated before, local methods are often more robust in the case of noise, while global techniques yield dense flow field. Bruhn et al. [19] propose a method that combines important advantages of local and global approaches and thus yields dense flow fields that are robust against noise. By inserting Eq. (2.60) into (2.61) we get

$$\mathcal{J}_{B}(\boldsymbol{u}) = \int_{\Omega} \mathbf{D}_{LK}(\mathcal{I}, \boldsymbol{u})^2 d\boldsymbol{x} + \alpha \int_{\Omega} \mathbf{S}(\boldsymbol{u}) d\boldsymbol{x} . \qquad (2.65)$$

In addition, they add an L_1-like penalizing function ψ to the individual terms in Eq. (2.65)

$$\mathcal{J}_{B}(\boldsymbol{u}) = \int_{\Omega} \psi_1(\mathbf{D}_{LK}(\mathcal{I}, \boldsymbol{u})^2) d\boldsymbol{x} + \alpha \int_{\Omega} \psi_2(\mathbf{S}(\boldsymbol{u})) d\boldsymbol{x} . \qquad (2.66)$$

A possible choice for ψ functions is given in Eq. (2.6), and ψ_1 and ψ_2 vary only in the choice of the parameter β. From a statistical viewpoint this can be regarded as applying methods from robust statistics where outliers are penalized less severely than in quadratic approaches. In general, such methods give better results at locations with flow discontinuities.

In a variety of applications the fundamental brightness constancy constraint in Eq. (2.53) may not apply. In the literature several alternatives have thus been proposed. One possibility is to demand constancy of image gradient or gradient magnitude. Other options include higher-order derivatives like the Hessian, Laplacian, or the determinant of the Hessian, photometric invariants, and texture features. Multiple features can also be combined towards complex constancy constraints (see [135] for an overview). In addition to the general development in computer vision, special attention has also been given to novel approaches motivated by medical imaging, e.g., [126].

While the accuracy of optical flow algorithms has improved steadily, the typical formulation has changed little since the seminal work of Horn and Schunck [64]. By means of a thorough analysis Sun et al. [125] attempt to uncover the "secrets" that have made recent advances possible. They analyze how the objective function, the optimization method, and modern implementation practices influence the accuracy. It is found that classical optical flow formulations perform surprisingly well when combined with modern optimization and implementation techniques (in particular, median filtering of intermediate flow fields during optimization).

2.2.4 Mass-Preserving Optical Flow

The aforementioned optical flow methods are all based on the brightness constancy constraint given in Eq. (2.53). However, this condition is not fulfilled in some imaging modalities, e.g., PET, due to partial volume effects, cf. Fig. 1.11. For such cases an optical flow method independent of this constraint is required.

As the total brightness of an organ can be considered constant for the duration of the image formation process, the continuity equation for the conservation of the total mass can be used as an alternative model, representing a Mass Preserving Optical Flow (MPOF) method [33]. The continuity equation for mass conservation is given as [10, 31]

$$\nabla \cdot (\mathcal{I}\boldsymbol{u}) = 0 \, , \tag{2.67}$$

where $\nabla \cdot$ is the divergence. Again, a functional can be defined based on Eq. (2.67) and minimized to get the optical flow estimate

$$\mathcal{J}(\boldsymbol{u}) := \int_{\Omega} (\nabla \cdot (\mathcal{I}\boldsymbol{u}))^2 d\boldsymbol{x} \overset{!}{=} \min \, . \tag{2.68}$$

Definition 2.12 (D_{mp} – Data term for mass-preserving optical flow). For two images $\mathcal{I}(x,t)$ and $\mathcal{I}(x,t+1)$ and a deformation (or velocity) field u the *data term for mass-preserving optical flow* is defined as

$$\mathbf{D}_{mp}(\mathcal{I},u) = \nabla \cdot (\mathcal{I}u)$$
$$= \mathcal{I}_x u + \mathcal{I}_y v + \mathcal{I}_z w + \mathcal{I}(u_x + v_y + w_z) + \mathcal{I}_t . \qquad (2.69)$$

As usual a regularization term is added to the functional, e.g., the diffusion regularization term of the Horn-Shunck method in Eq. (2.62). The mass-preserving optical flow functional to be minimized is therefore

$$\mathcal{J}_{mp}(u) = \int_\Omega \mathbf{D}_{mp}(\mathcal{I},u)^2 dx + \alpha \int_\Omega \mathbf{S}(u)dx , \qquad (2.70)$$

where α is the regularization parameter. The corresponding Euler-Lagrange equations are given by

$$0 = \mathbf{D}_x \mathcal{I} + \alpha \Delta u ,$$
$$0 = \mathbf{D}_y \mathcal{I} + \alpha \Delta v , \qquad (2.71)$$
$$0 = \mathbf{D}_z \mathcal{I} + \alpha \Delta w ,$$

where $\mathbf{D}_x, \mathbf{D}_y, \mathbf{D}_z$ are the derivatives of $\mathbf{D}_{mp}$ in the corresponding directions. Solving this system leads to the following iterative scheme

$$u^{k+1} = u^k + \mathbf{D}_x \mathcal{I} + \alpha \Delta u ,$$
$$v^{k+1} = v^k + \mathbf{D}_y \mathcal{I} + \alpha \Delta v , \qquad (2.72)$$
$$w^{k+1} = w^k + \mathbf{D}_z \mathcal{I} + \alpha \Delta w .$$

Algorithm 2.4 Mass-preserving optical flow method

Input: Images $\mathcal{I}(x,t)$ and $\mathcal{I}(x,t+1)$
Output: Motion estimate u (for all voxels)
   initialize u for all voxels, e.g., null vector
   while change in u > threshold **do**
      for each voxel x **do**
         compute $u(x)$ as given in Eqs. (2.72)
      end for
   end while

As shown above in Sect. 2.2.3, the motion discontinuities can be better modeled if an L_1-like penelization term is applied. Using the aforementioned function ψ in Eq. (2.6) we get

$$\mathcal{J}_{mpn}(u) = \int_\Omega \psi_1(\mathbf{D}_{mp}(\mathcal{I}, u)^2)dx + \alpha \int_\Omega \psi_2(\mathbf{S}(u))dx \,, \qquad (2.73)$$

where ψ_1 and ψ_2 vary only in the choice of the parameter β in Eq. (2.6). The corresponding Euler-Lagrange equations can be found in [37]. The optical flow can be estimated by using an iterative scheme similar to that given above in Algorithm 2.4 for the quadratic case.

2.2.5 Multi-level Optimization

As in the case of image registration, the proposed optical flow methods should be applied in a multi-level framework to avoid local minima during optimization, cf. Sect. 2.1.5. The multi-level framework becomes particularly important for optical flow methods as it allows the treatment of large motion with the Taylor approximation, which only holds for small displacements. The motion is thus calculated on a coarse level, where it is still small in terms of voxel size. Starting at the lowest level we get a rough estimate of the flow vectors. These vectors are prolonged (interpolated) to the next higher level. On that level the original template image is interpolated with the current transformation. Again, the flow is estimated, but on the finer resolution, to figure out the residual motion. This process is repeated until the maximal resolution is reached.

As the motion vectors are estimated with the mass-preserving motion model, the transformation of the template image needs to be mass-preserving as well. The approximation in Eq. (2.67) is used in [33] for the mass-preserving transformation of the template image. For this approximation the time derivative in the equation is calculated as $\mathcal{I}_t = \mathcal{T} - \mathcal{R}$. As the optical flow u in Eq. (2.67) is known after motion estimation the motion corrected image can be calculated according to

$$\mathcal{T}^{MC}(x) = \mathcal{T}(x) + \nabla \cdot (\mathcal{T}(x)u(x)) \,, \, \forall x \in \Omega \,. \qquad (2.74)$$

This equation is accurate for small displacements. However, this assumption does not hold for potentially large non-linear cardiac displacements. A better, non-approximated, method is to use the mass-preserving transformation model in Definition 2.11 based on the exact computation of the Jacobian determinant. Accordingly, the motion corrected image is calculated as

$$\mathcal{T}^{MC}(x) = \mathcal{T}(x + u(x)) \cdot \det(\nabla(x + u(x))) \,, \, \forall x \in \Omega \,. \qquad (2.75)$$

This image is then used as the template image for the next level. The proceeding is summarized in Algorithm 2.5.

Algorithm 2.5 Mass-preserving multi-level optical flow

Input: Template image $\mathcal{T}\ (=\mathcal{I}(\boldsymbol{x},t))$ and reference image $\mathcal{R}\ (=\mathcal{I}(\boldsymbol{x},t+1))$
Output: Motion estimate $\boldsymbol{u}$ (for all voxels)
   initialize $\boldsymbol{u}_{\mathrm{minLevel}}$ for all voxels, e.g., null vector
   for level $=$ minLevel $\rightarrow$ maxLevel **do**
     $\mathcal{R}_{\mathrm{level}} \leftarrow \mathcal{R}$ // down-sampling
     $\mathcal{T}_{\mathrm{level}} \overset{u}{\leftarrow} \mathcal{T}$ // apply motion with mass-preservation $\mathcal{M}^{\mathrm{MP}}(\mathcal{T},\boldsymbol{x}+\boldsymbol{u}(\boldsymbol{x}))$ & down-sampling
               // NOTE: the exact computation of the Jacobian is used
     $\boldsymbol{u}_{\mathrm{level}} \leftarrow \mathrm{argmin}\mathcal{J}_{\mathrm{mp}}(\boldsymbol{u}_{\mathrm{level}})$ // update motion by minimizing the functional
     if level $<$ maxLevel **then**
       $\boldsymbol{u}_{\mathrm{level}+1} \leftarrow \boldsymbol{u}_{\mathrm{level}}$ // prolongate motion to next level
     end if
   end for
   $\boldsymbol{u} \leftarrow \boldsymbol{u}_{\mathrm{maxLevel}}$ // output final motion estimate

---

2.2.6 Results

The MPOF approach is applied to the same XCAT software phantom data as described in Sect. 2.1.6 in connection with the VAMPIRE approach. The results of MPOF are visualized in Fig. 2.9 for the same slice used in Figs. 2.7 and 2.8. The gate in maximum inspiration and systole is chosen here as the template image $\mathcal{T}$ (shown in Fig. 2.9a), as it is the most different gate compared to the reference image $\mathcal{R}$ in maximum expiration and diastole (shown in Fig. 2.9b). Additionally, the transformed template image according to the estimated transformation, i.e., $\mathcal{M}^{\mathrm{MP}}(\mathcal{T},\boldsymbol{y}_{\mathrm{OF}})$, and a vector plot are given in Fig. 2.9c, d. Some quantitative numbers based on the ground-truth transformation will be given at the end of following Sect. 2.3.

2.3 Comparison and Evaluation

In the previous sections we have seen two different approaches to mass-preserving motion estimation. The variant based on image registration is given in Sect. 2.1.4 and the optical flow variant is derived in Sect. 2.2.4. Technically, optical flow and image registration approaches provide different approaches to motion estimation. On the one hand, the image registration framework simplifies the incorporation of physically meaningful regularization like (non-linear) hyperelasticity. On the other hand, optical flow has also several advantages as it is, e.g., computationally efficient due to the linear Taylor approximation. Both approaches have in common that they are generally well understood. That means that they are versatile with a variety of different possible configurations (e.g., intensity or gradient distance measures).

One of the main differences between image registration and optical flow, as presented in this book, is the numerical realization. While image registration is based on a discretize-then-optimize strategy, optical flow follows an optimize-then-discretize strategy. The optimization in the case of optical flow includes a Taylor approximation whereas image registration relies on the exact computation of all its components. The Taylor approximation makes, e.g., the incorporation of non-linear hyperelastic regularization into the optical flow functional in Eq. (2.70) challenging. Hyperelasticity would thus transform into something like linear elasticity, which is only suitable for small deformations.

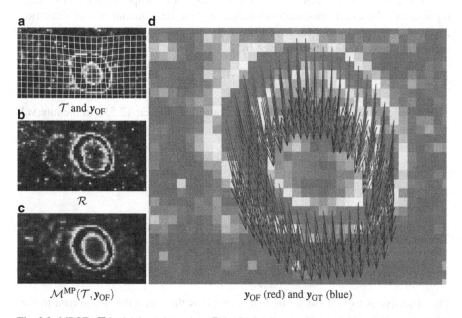

Fig. 2.9 MPOF: $\mathcal{T}$ in (**a**) is registered to $\mathcal{R}$ in (**b**) leading to the overlaid transformation grid in (**a**). The transformed template image is shown in (**c**). A magnification with a comparison of the estimated vectors (*red*) and the ground-truth vectors (*blue*) is shown in (**d**). (Colored figures are only available in the online version.)

2.3.1 Comparison

Despite the fundamental differences, the basic idea of MPOF and VAMPIRE is the same. Hence, we will derive the mass-preserving optical flow equations from the VAMPIRE model in the following. For this purpose, let us recall the concept of mass-preservation as introduced in Sect. 2.1.4. The idea of mass-preserving image registration is the preservation of the total intensity of an image due to a transformation model $\mathcal{M}$

$$\int_{\mathbf{y}(\Omega)} \mathcal{T}(\mathbf{x}) d\mathbf{x} = \int_{\Omega} \mathcal{M}(\mathcal{T}, \mathbf{y}(\mathbf{x})) \, d\mathbf{x} \,, \tag{2.76}$$

which is exactly given by the integration by substitution theorem for multiple variables

$$\int_{\mathbf{y}(\Omega)} \mathcal{T}(\mathbf{x}) d\mathbf{x} = \int_{\Omega} \mathcal{T}(\mathbf{y}(\mathbf{x})) \, \det(\nabla \mathbf{y}(\mathbf{x})) \, d\mathbf{x} \,. \tag{2.77}$$

This is the same equation that was used for the derivation of VAMPIRE in Eq. (2.45). Since optical flow is generally speaking a Taylor approximation of image registration, the exact computation of the Jacobian determinant in the VAMPIRE approach is approximated for MPOF as well. The transformation model for mass-preserving image registration is given by

$$\mathcal{M}^{\text{MP}}(\mathcal{T}, \mathbf{y}) = (\mathcal{T} \circ \mathbf{y}) \cdot \det(\nabla \mathbf{y}) \,. \tag{2.78}$$

We will restrict the time variable t of $\mathcal{I}$, introduced in Eq. (2.53), to the interval $[0,1]$ to make the transition from image registration to optical flow

$$\mathcal{I}(\mathbf{x}, t) : \mathbb{R}^3 \times [0,1] \to \mathbb{R} \text{ with}$$
$$\mathcal{I}(\cdot, 0) = \mathcal{T} \text{ and} \tag{2.79}$$
$$\mathcal{I}(\cdot, 1) = \mathcal{R} \,.$$

The time variable is also introduced for the corresponding transformations

$$\mathbf{y}(\mathbf{x}, t) : \mathbb{R}^3 \times [0,1] \to \mathbb{R}^3 \,. \tag{2.80}$$

The objective is to find the set of transformations that align the image data to the reference frame

$$\mathcal{I}(\mathbf{y}(\cdot, t), t) \stackrel{!}{=} \mathcal{R} = \mathcal{I}(\mathbf{x}, 1) \,, \forall \mathbf{x} \in [0,1] \,. \tag{2.81}$$

Note that $\mathbf{y}(\cdot, 1)$ is the identity transformation.

The equation known from image registration

$$\int_{\Omega} \mathcal{T}(\mathbf{y}(\mathbf{x})) \cdot \det(\nabla \mathbf{y}(\mathbf{x})) \, d\mathbf{x} \tag{2.82}$$

at time t now reads

$$\int_{\Omega} \mathcal{I}(\mathbf{y}(\mathbf{x}, t), t) \cdot \det(\nabla \mathbf{y}(\mathbf{x}, t)) \, d\mathbf{x} \,. \tag{2.83}$$

According to [10] we compute the temporal derivative

$$\int_\Omega \frac{\delta}{\delta t} \left(\mathcal{I}(\boldsymbol{y}(\boldsymbol{x},t),t) \cdot \det(\nabla \boldsymbol{y}(\boldsymbol{x},t)) \right) d\boldsymbol{x}, \tag{2.84}$$

which yields (approximately)

$$\int_\Omega \left(\nabla \mathcal{I}(\boldsymbol{y}(\boldsymbol{x},t),t) \cdot \frac{\delta}{\delta t}(\boldsymbol{y}(\boldsymbol{x},t)) + \mathcal{I}(\boldsymbol{y}(\boldsymbol{x},t),t) \cdot \left(\nabla \cdot \frac{\delta}{\delta t}(\boldsymbol{y}(\boldsymbol{x},t)) \right) \right) \det(\nabla \boldsymbol{y}(\boldsymbol{x},t)) \, d\boldsymbol{x}, \tag{2.85}$$

by using the chain rule and the approximation

$$\frac{\delta}{\delta t} \det(\nabla \boldsymbol{y}(\boldsymbol{x},t)) \approx \left(\nabla \cdot \frac{\delta}{\delta t}(\boldsymbol{y}(\boldsymbol{x},t)) \right) \det(\nabla \boldsymbol{y}(\boldsymbol{x},t)). \tag{2.86}$$

Like in standard optical flow we set the integral in Eq. (2.85) equal to zero and get

$$0 = (\nabla \mathcal{I})^T \boldsymbol{u} + \mathcal{I}_t + \mathcal{I} \nabla \cdot \boldsymbol{u} \tag{2.87}$$

$$\Longleftrightarrow 0 = \nabla \cdot (\mathcal{I}\boldsymbol{u}) + \mathcal{I}_t, \tag{2.88}$$

where $\boldsymbol{u}^T = \left(\frac{\delta}{\delta t}\boldsymbol{y}_x(\boldsymbol{x},t), \frac{\delta}{\delta t}\boldsymbol{y}_y(\boldsymbol{x},t), \frac{\delta}{\delta t}\boldsymbol{y}_z(\boldsymbol{x},t) \right) =: (u,v,w)$ is the velocity. As we are only dealing with the registration of two images, $\mathcal{I}$ consists only of two images ($\mathcal{T}$ and $\mathcal{R}$) and $\boldsymbol{u}$ is reduced to one velocity field connecting these two images. This finally leads to the data term for mass-preserving optical flow that we know from Definition 2.12.

One important assumption of both, optical flow and image registration, is a positive Jacobian determinant, i.e., $\det(\nabla \boldsymbol{y}) > 0$. As the exact values of the Jacobian determinant are used for image registration, this can be ensured by simply disallowing negative values. However, optical flow requires more effort to guarantee diffeomorphic transformations as, e.g., proposed by Yang et al. [137]. The idea is to restrict the motion update to a vector less than 0.4 voxel which prevents foldings and preserves diffeomorphic motion estimates. This, however, might reduce the convergence speed of the overall algorithm. In practice we even observe a similar run-time compared to image registration where in each Gauss-Newton iteration a large and complicated linear system needs to be solved. Another approach by Vercauteren et al. [132] uses an approximation of the exponential of the deformation to ensure diffeomorphisms. As the proposed implementation is only based on an approximation of the exponential of the deformation it finally gives no real guarantee for $\det(\nabla \boldsymbol{y}) > 0$ [137].

In conclusion, mass-preserving optical flow and mass-preserving image registration are based on the same assumption, i.e., preservation of the overall radioactivity. Both approaches just differ in their technical realization. On experimental and clinical data we could show that both approaches yield satisfying (i.e., realistic) results with comparable accuracy for PET motion correction, see [37, 51] and the evaluation at the end of this section. It is thus difficult to give preference to one particular method in practice for all applications. The discussion above is intended to provide some orientation in the reader's decision-making process for one method. In order to give more assistance we perform a quantitative evaluation of both methods in the following.

2.3.2   Evaluation

The following evaluation is carried out on *software phantom data* and *patient data*. While the analysis based on the software phantom data is performed to quantitatively compare the image registration and optical flow based approaches, the patient study shows the general clinical applicability of the proposed methods.

2.3.2.1   Software Phantom Data

The images of the software phantom evaluation are based on the results presented in Fig. 2.8 for VAMPIRE and Fig. 2.9 for MPOF. More information about the XCAT software phantom data and in particular the image generation process can be found in Sect. 2.1.6.

Results

For a visual comparison we show some results of the proposed methods for motion estimation in Fig. 2.10. Cardiac slices are shown for a single gate in Fig. 2.10a for the reference gate $\mathcal{R}$, showing a high noise level. The combination of all available gates, representing a reconstruction without any motion correction, is given in Fig. 2.10b. This image features severe motion induced artifacts compared to the reference gate $\mathcal{R}$, thus demanding for motion correction techniques. However, the SNR is significantly higher compared to the single gate in Fig. 2.10a. The combination of all single gates using the ground-truth motion information, provided by XCAT, can be found in Fig. 2.10c. Accordingly, this image represents the best possible, and thus desired, image quality as it combines the high SNR of Fig. 2.10b and the reduced motion of Fig. 2.10a. The resulting images based on estimated motion can be found in Fig. 2.10d for the image registration based SAD VAMPIRE approach and in Fig. 2.10e for the MPOF approach. The image quality of both approaches is comparable with the image based on the ground-truth motion in Fig. 2.10c.

Validation

The results which are shown in Fig. 2.10 and the underlying motion estimates are quantitatively evaluated. The results are given in Table 2.1. The endpoint error e is used to determine the Euclidean distance of the estimated and the ground-truth deformation. For two transformations $\boldsymbol{y}_1, \boldsymbol{y}_2 : \mathbb{R}^3 \to \mathbb{R}^3$ and a non-empty set $\Omega \subset \mathbb{R}^3$ the endpoint error is defined as

$$e(\boldsymbol{y}_1, \boldsymbol{y}_2) := \frac{1}{|\Omega|} \int_\Omega |\boldsymbol{y}_1(\boldsymbol{x}) - \boldsymbol{y}_2(\boldsymbol{x})| d\boldsymbol{x}, \tag{2.89}$$

where $|\Omega| := \int_\Omega d\boldsymbol{x}$ and for vectors $|\cdot|$ is the Euclidean norm. The values given in the table are averaged values over all gates. The maximum endpoint error is considered to analyze the worst case of the transformation mismatch and is defined as

$$e^{\max}(\boldsymbol{y}_1, \boldsymbol{y}_2) := \max_{\boldsymbol{x} \in \Omega} |\boldsymbol{y}_1(\boldsymbol{x}) - \boldsymbol{y}_2(\boldsymbol{x})|. \tag{2.90}$$

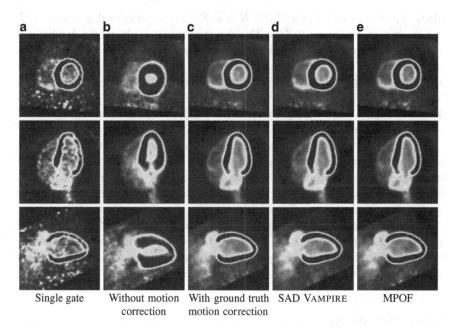

| a | b | c | d | e |

Single gate Without motion With ground truth SAD VAMPIRE MPOF
correction motion correction

Fig. 2.10 The cardiac planes (from *top* to *bottom*: SA, HLA, and VLA) are shown for the single reference gate $\mathcal{R}$ in (**a**) out of a 5×5 dual gating. The combination of all gates without any motion correction can be seen in (**b**). Motion artifacts in terms of blurring can be clearly seen. The motion corrected image based on the ground-truth motion is shown in (**c**). The image shows a reduced blurring, e.g., in the blood pool. The results of the image registration based SAD VAMPIRE approach and the optical flow based MPOF approach are shown in (**d**) and (**e**). The image quality of the proposed VAMPIRE and MPOF approach is comparable to the best possible result based on ground-truth motion and considerably better than the resulting image without any motion correction. All images are corrected for attenuation

The values given in the table denote the maximum error over all dual gates. The transformation's regularity is analyzed via the range of the Jacobian map

$$\left[\min_{x\in\Omega}\{\det(\nabla y(x))\}\ ,\ \max_{x\in\Omega}\{\det(\nabla y(x))\}\right].\qquad(2.91)$$

Orientation preserving and diffeomorphic transformations, i.e., transformations free of foldings, can be assured by controlling the maximum decrease or increase of a voxel's volume or intensity. Finite values greater than 0 represent appropriate values for the Jacobian map. A value of 1 indicates no volume change.

The Normalized Cross-Correlation (NCC) measure is suitable for general intensity-based validation. For two images $\mathcal{T}:\Omega\to\mathbb{R}$ and $\mathcal{R}:\Omega\to\mathbb{R}$ on a domain $\Omega\subset\mathbb{R}^3$ the NCC is defined as

$$\mathrm{NCC}(\mathcal{T},\mathcal{R}):=\frac{\int_\Omega \mathcal{T}_\mu(x)\mathcal{R}_\mu(x)\,dx}{\sqrt{\int_\Omega \mathcal{T}_\mu(x)^2\,dx}\sqrt{\int_\Omega \mathcal{R}_\mu(x)^2\,dx}}\ ,\qquad(2.92)$$

where $\mathcal{T}_\mu=\mathcal{T}-\mu(\mathcal{T})$ and $\mathcal{R}_\mu=\mathcal{R}-\mu(\mathcal{R})$ are the unbiased versions of $\mathcal{T}$ and $\mathcal{R}$. For an image $\mathcal{I}$, $\mu(\mathcal{I})$ is the expected value. It should be emphasized that the validation based on image intensities can only give certain hints on the accuracy of the registration process. Indeed, it was shown in [115] that even inaccurate registration results can produce good scores on intensity-based measures. Accordingly, the combination with ground-truth transformation-based measures discussed before is mandatory. In Table 2.1 $\mathrm{NCC}(\mathcal{T},\mathcal{R})$ represents the similarity before motion correction and $\mathrm{NCC}(\mathcal{M}^{\mathrm{MP}}(\mathcal{T},y),\mathcal{R})$ after motion correction.

The values in Table 2.1 indicate that all proposed methods have a comparable accuracy. The average endpoint errors e and the maximum endpoint errors $e^{\max}$ are very close to each other and reveal a sub-voxel accuracy for each method, given a voxel size of 3.375 mm. The Jacobian range demonstrates that all results are diffeomorphic and thus free of foldings. The correlation values also increase after motion correction. The reason why the values for $\mathrm{NCC}(\mathcal{M}^{\mathrm{MP}}(\mathcal{T},y),\mathcal{R})$ after motion correction are not 1 is that the random noise in the image prevents a perfect match. With other words, a too high correlation would indicate an unwanted match of the random noise in the images during motion estimation.

2.3.2.2   Patient Data

In Fig. 1.1 we have already seen the effect of motion correction on real patient data as a motivation. The shown data is part of a set of 21 patients (19 male, 2 female; between 37 and 76 years old) with known coronary artery disease. One hour after injection of ^{18}F-FDG (4 MBq/kg) a 20 min list mode scan was acquired for evaluation of myocardial viability prior to revascularization. All patients underwent a hyperinsulinemic euglycemic clamp technique before and during the scan to enhance FDG uptake in the heart. In addition, β-blockers were administered to all

Table 2.1 Evaluation of SSD VAMPIRE, SAD VAMPIRE, and MPOF based on common validation criteria. The definitions of the validation criteria are given in this section. The numbers for $e(\boldsymbol{y}, \boldsymbol{y}_{GT})$ and NCC are average values over all 25 dual gates. The range of the Jacobian map represents the global minimum and maximum for all images. The maximum end-point error is also the global maximum error for all images

	SSD VAMPIRE	SAD VAMPIRE	MPOF
$e(\boldsymbol{y}, \boldsymbol{y}_{GT})$	1.50 mm	1.46 mm	1.45 mm
$e^{\max}(\boldsymbol{y}, \boldsymbol{y}_{GT})$	8.19 mm	6.00 mm	5.64 mm
$\min_{\boldsymbol{x}}\{\det(\nabla \boldsymbol{y}(\boldsymbol{x}))\}$	0.64	0.58	0.39
$\max_{\boldsymbol{x}}\{\det(\nabla \boldsymbol{y}(\boldsymbol{x}))\}$	1.19	1.44	1.45
$\text{NCC}(\mathcal{T}, \mathcal{R})$	0.61	0.61	0.61
$\text{NCC}(\mathcal{M}^{\text{MP}}(\mathcal{T}, \boldsymbol{y}), \mathcal{R})$	0.87	0.88	0.88

patients to lower and keep constant the heart rate during examination. All scans were performed on a Siemens Biograph^{TM} Sensation 16 PET/CT scanner (Siemens Medical Solution) with a spatial resolution of around 6–7 mm [41]. During list mode acquisition an ECG signal was recorded for cardiac gating.

A phase-based cardiac gating with variable widths throughout all cycles and equal widths within each cycle is performed. The respiratory signals are estimated on basis of list mode data without auxiliary measurements [23]. An amplitude-based gating is applied to the respiratory signal, deduced from changes in the center of mass. For each of the 21 patients we choose 25 gates (five respiratory and five cardiac gates).

Image reconstruction is performed with the 3D EM software EMRECON [77,78]. Twenty iterations with one subset are chosen. The output images are sampled with $175 \times 175 \times 47$ voxels. Given an isotropic voxel size of 3.375 mm, this results in a Field Of View (FOV) of $590.625 \times 590.625 \times 158.625$ mm. To prevent the attenuation correction artifacts discussed above, cf. [34], motion correction is performed on data that is not corrected for attenuation during reconstruction.

Results

We have seen in Table 2.1 that the performance of VAMPIRE and MPOF is comparable in practice. Thus we only show results from one method in the following analysis. Specifically, the presented results were generated with VAMPIRE and the SSD distance measure. We chose the gate in mid-expiration and diastole as our reference image $\mathcal{R}$ as diastole is the most common cardiac phase and the maximum motion of mid-expiration to all other respiratory phases is on average the smallest. We set the hyperelastic regularization parameters in Eq. (2.17) to $\alpha_l = 5$, $\alpha_a = 1$, and $\alpha_v = 10$ according to [51].

The effects of motion correction are illustrated for one patient in Fig. 2.11. The reference phase $\mathcal{R}$ in mid-expiration and diastole is shown in Fig. 2.11a. One particular template image $\mathcal{T}$ out of the 24 remaining gates is shown in Fig. 2.11b. We chose the gate in maximum inspiration and systole which is very dissimilar to $\mathcal{R}$. The grid representing the estimated transformation is overlaid on $\mathcal{T}$. Volume changes induced by this transformation are visualized in Fig. 2.11c. After applying the estimated transformation to $\mathcal{T}$ with the mass-preserving transformation model we obtain the image shown in Fig. 2.11d. The absolute difference images before and after applying the estimated transformation are given in Fig. 2.11e, f. Combining all 25 motion corrected gates yields the final image in Fig. 2.11g. A clear reduction of motion induced blurring can be observed compared to the image without motion correction in Fig. 2.11h.

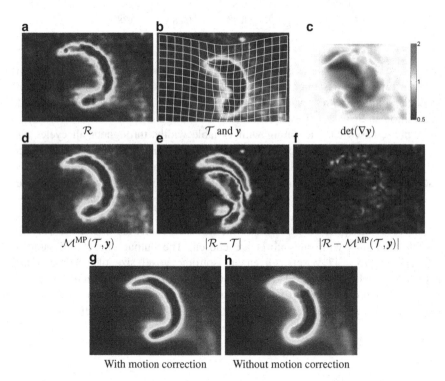

Fig. 2.11 Effects of motion correction illustrated for one patient. (**b**) is registered to $\mathcal{R}$ (**a**) using VAMPIRE resulting in (**d**). The absolute difference image before (**e**) and after motion correction (**f**) illustrate the accuracy. The estimated transformation $\mathbf{y}$ (**b**) is smooth and free of foldings which can also be seen at the plot of the Jacobian map (**c**). The logarithmic color map ranges from 0.5 (*blue*) over 1 (*white*) to 2 (*red*). The *bottom row* shows the final image with (**g**) and without (**h**) motion correction. (The images are taken from [51]. © 2011 IEEE. Colored figures are only available in the online version.)

Validation

We perform a validation of the patient data based on the range of the Jacobian determinant and the NCC defined in Eqs. (2.91) and (2.92). The minimum of all Jacobian maps (for all patients and all gates) is 0.340 and the maximum is 2.375. As no negative or too large values appear we can ensure that no unwanted foldings occur in the estimated transformations. For the NCC we can observe an improvement from 0.88 ± 0.07 to 0.97 ± 0.002 on average across all patients. For the most challenging gates in relation to the reference gate, i.e., heart in systole and heart in maximum inspiration, we found an increase from 0.80 ± 0.06 to 0.97 ± 0.001 and 0.79 ± 0.06 to 0.97 ± 0.002, respectively. Figure 2.12 illustrates the average NCC values for the cardiac and respiratory phases individually. The two most challenging phases are gate two in Fig. 2.12a, representing the systole, and gate five in Fig. 2.12b, representing the gate in maximum inspiration.

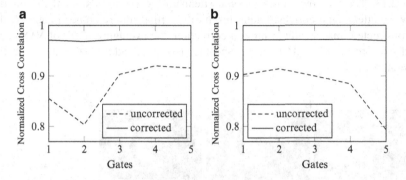

Fig. 2.12 The average NCC before and after motion correction is plotted for all cardiac (**a**) and respiratory (**b**) gates for the patient data (The plots are taken from [51]. © 2011 IEEE)

Attenuation Correction

Additional corrections like scatter and attenuation correction are necessary to make the presented results quantitative [38]. As attenuation correction is not the focus of this chapter we give only a short outlook. According to the method proposed by Bai and Brady [8] we perform an image-based attenuation correction. The idea of their attenuation correction approach is to reconstruct the PET reference gate $\mathcal{R}$ twice – once *with* attenuation correction ($\mathcal{R}^{AC}$, AC = Attenuation Corrected) and once *without* ($\mathcal{R}^{NAC}$, NAC = Non-Attenuation Corrected). Hence, an additional CT scan that matches the reference PET gate $\mathcal{R}$ is required. The Attenuation Coefficient Factor (ACF) image $\mathcal{I}^{ACF} = \frac{\mathcal{R}^{AC}}{\mathcal{R}^{NAC}}$ of the two reference images is computed. For the reference gate it holds

$$\mathcal{R}^{\text{AC}} = \mathcal{I}^{\text{ACF}} \cdot \mathcal{R}^{\text{NAC}} = \frac{\mathcal{R}^{\text{AC}}}{\mathcal{R}^{\text{NAC}}} \cdot \mathcal{R}^{\text{NAC}} . \tag{2.93}$$

As the average image

$$\mathcal{T}_{\text{avg}} = \mathcal{T}_{\text{avg}}^{\text{NAC}} = \frac{1}{25} \sum_{r=1}^{5} \sum_{c=1}^{5} \mathcal{M}^{\text{MP}}(\mathcal{T}_r^c, \boldsymbol{y}_r^c) \tag{2.94}$$

matches the reference phase, we can approximate the attenuation corrected version through

$$\mathcal{T}_{\text{avg}}^{\text{AC}} = \mathcal{I}^{\text{ACF}} \cdot \mathcal{T}_{\text{avg}}^{\text{NAC}} = \frac{\mathcal{R}^{\text{AC}}}{\mathcal{R}^{\text{NAC}}} \cdot \mathcal{T}_{\text{avg}}^{\text{NAC}} = \mathcal{R}^{\text{AC}} \cdot \frac{\mathcal{T}_{\text{avg}}^{\text{NAC}}}{\mathcal{R}^{\text{NAC}}} . \tag{2.95}$$

The results of the patient data with attenuation correction are illustrated in Fig. 2.13. The top row shows the *non*-attenuation corrected data and the middle row the attenuation corrected data. From left to right: the reference image $\mathcal{R}$, the reconstructed image without motion correction, the averaging result of VAMPIRE, and line profiles. The ACF image and the μ-map are additionally shown in the bottom row.

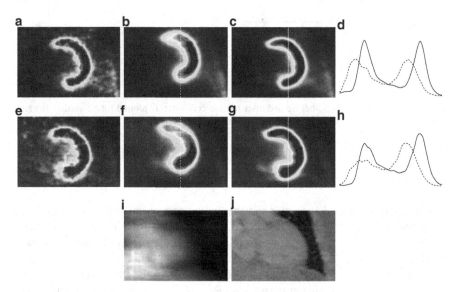

Fig. 2.13 Comparison of Non-Attenuation Corrected (NAC) and Attenuation Corrected (AC) patient data. (**a**) $\mathcal{R}^{\text{NAC}}$ (**b**) No MC, NAC (**c**) VAMPIRE, NAC (**d**) Line profiles NAC (**e**) $\mathcal{R}^{\text{AC}}$ (**f**) No MC, AC (**g**) VAMPIRE, AC (**h**) Line profiles AC (**i**) ACF image $\mathcal{I}^{\text{ACF}}$ (**j**) μ-map

The main message of Fig. 2.13 is that the application of attenuation correction may induce severe artifacts to cardiac PET data which can be overcome by our proposed motion estimation and motion correction approaches. The mentioned artifacts can be observed in the upper region of the left ventricle in Fig. 2.13f. The radioactivity distribution is strongly underestimated due to the misalignment of the μ-map in Fig. 2.13j and the PET data in Fig. 2.13b. However, as attenuation correction is essential for quantitative evaluations we can choose the reference image $\mathcal{R}$ as the respiratory and cardiac phase representing the same motion state as the μ-map and perform motion correction. The resulting image with motion correction and attenuation correction in Fig. 2.13g is no longer affected by the artifacts present in Fig. 2.13f and can thus be used for further quantitative clinical evaluations.

Chapter 3
Motion Correction

In the previous chapter we have seen tailored methods for the estimation of motion between gates representing different motion states. Based on this knowledge, we eliminate motion induced image artifacts in a subsequent correction step. In this chapter, we give an overview of strategies for motion correction. The presented correction techniques vary between methods which rely on already available motion information (e.g., averaging) and methods that incorporate motion estimation into the correction procedure (e.g., joint reconstruction of image and motion). In this context, we particularly introduce advanced motion correction pipelines for dual gated PET which efficiently combine motion estimation and elimination.

3.1 Motion Correction Strategies

We already introduced the basic concept of motion correction in Sect. 1.5, focusing mainly on motion correction schemes based on gating with subsequent motion estimation and correction. A more detailed discussion on these approaches is given in the following.

To reduce motion and its impact on further analysis in thoracic PET, several approaches were proposed recently. Unlike the more sophisticated approaches that try to estimate motion and subsequently correct for it, optimized gating approaches have recently been introduced in clinical diagnostics, called *optimal gating*. Almost all other approaches have in common that motion is estimated on the basis of PET data instead of, e.g., gated CT images, in order to keep the radiation burden as low as possible. They can be classified into the four groups introduced in Sect. 1.5.1 plus the optimal gating strategy:

1. Optimal gating
2. Averaging of aligned images

© The Author(s) 2015
F. Gigengack et al., *Motion Correction in Thoracic Positron Emission Tomography*,
SpringerBriefs in Electrical and Computer Engineering,
DOI 10.1007/978-3-319-08392-6_3

3. Motion compensated re-reconstruction
4. Event rebinning
5. Joint reconstruction of image and motion

3.1.1   Optimal Gating

In contrast to cardiac motion induced by myocardial contraction, respiratory motion has a quite irregular pattern. Most of the time, the thorax is resting at the expiration phase, whereas the inspiration phase is often relatively short. Recently, a new amplitude-based gating approach, called *optimal gating*, was introduced by van Elmpt et al. [131] that defines the maximum time phase at end-expiration where the motion is minimal. Therefore, a histogram is formed of the respiratory signals, acquired during the list mode PET scan, and converted to a cumulative distribution function. On this function, a lower and upper level is determined that forces the total sensitivity to equal to a certain percentage (e.g., 35 %) of the acquired breathing signals. This percentage is called the *optimal gating yield*.

Although most of the acquired data (e.g., 65 %) is discarded in performing optimal gating leading to noisier images, this approach provides a robust method of motion reduction. It could be demonstrated that optimal gating is a user-friendly respiratory gating method to increase detectability and quantification of upper abdominal lesions compared to conventional acquisition techniques [130].

3.1.2   Averaging of Aligned Images

After gating the acquired PET data, each gate is reconstructed individually and aligned to one designated reference gate. To overcome the problem of low SNRs, the aligned images are averaged (summed) afterwards. In the context of respiratory motion correction, Dawood et al. [34] propose an optical flow based approach and Bai et al. [6–8] use a regularized B-spline approach with a Markov random field regularizer. In the context of cardiac motion correction, Klein et al. [73, 75] propose a technique using 3D optical flow and model the myocardium as an elastic membrane. In their approach intensity modulations caused by cardiac motion (see Sect. 2.1.4) are not addressed. The averaging of aligned images is described in more detail in Sect. 3.2.1 of this book.

3.1.3   Motion Compensated Re-reconstruction

Similar to the averaging approach, gating is applied and each individually reconstructed gate is aligned to one assigned reference gate. The obtained motion information is incorporated into a subsequent re-reconstruction of the whole data set. The lines of response are adjusted according to the motion field which implies time-varying system matrices, see [46, 80, 111, 112] for respiratory motion correction approaches. Motion compensated re-reconstruction is also used in Sect. 3.2.3 in connection with the simplified motion correction pipeline.

3.1.4 Event Rebinning

The acquired list mode data is gated and each gate is reconstructed. Motion is estimated based on these reconstructed images. The initial list mode data is rebinned in a subsequent step by applying the transformation gained from the motion estimation step [79]. As only affine transformations are allowed, such methods can correct for respiratory motion (which is primarily locally rigid) to a certain extent but not for non-linear cardiac motion.

3.1.5 Joint Reconstruction of Image and Motion

In joint reconstruction, motion is estimated simultaneously to the reconstruction of the image [13, 14, 20, 68, 89, 121]. An objective function is optimized in two arguments: image and motion. Hence, only *one* image with the full statistics is reconstructed. A drawback of these approaches is the relatively high computational cost.

3.2 Motion Correction Pipelines for Dual Gated PET

As we have seen with the motion correction approaches discussed so far, motion is typically estimated between each gate and a certain reference gate (based on the motion estimation methods presented in Chap. 2) and eliminated subsequently in a gate-by-gate manner. This intuitive motion correction procedure is further described with the serial pipeline in Sect. 3.2.1 specifically for dual gated PET. However, dual gated PET offers more advanced opportunities for the correction step. In Sects. 3.2.2 and 3.2.3 we present pipelines for motion correction which efficiently combine motion estimation and motion correction. The key feature is thereby the decoupling of respiratory and cardiac motion. This means that respiratory and cardiac motion are estimated separately with intermediate correction steps. As a result, the presented simplified pipelines feature a reduced number of motion estimation steps with an increased robustness towards noise in each step.

3.2.1 Serial Pipeline

The core idea of the *serial pipeline* for motion correction in dual gated PET, as proposed in [51], is a sequential execution of the motion estimation and motion correction step. First, the whole $m \times n$ matrix of m respiratory and n cardiac images is built. The $m \times n$ matrix consists of the individual reconstructions of all dual PET gates. An example of a dual gating image matrix is given in Fig. 1.7. After choosing a particular reference phase, each of the $m \cdot n - 1$ remaining (template) images is registered to this reference phase with the methods described in Chap. 2. The motion correction step is performed by means of a subsequent averaging of the transformed (i.e., motion corrected) gates. In summary, this serial pipeline consists of the following steps:

1. Determination of the dual gating signal
2. Reconstruction of all dual gates   ($m \cdot n$ resulting images)
3. Dual motion estimation   ($m \cdot n - 1$ registration tasks)
4. Averaging of all motion corrected dual gates   (1 resulting image)

The steps of the serial pipeline are visualized in Fig. 3.1. This schematic illustration facilitates a comparison to the pipelines presented in the remainder of this chapter, cf. Figs. 3.2 and 3.3.

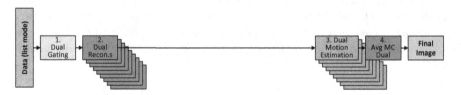

Fig. 3.1 Schematic illustration of the serial pipeline. All dual gates are reconstructed and used for a gate-by-gate motion estimation. Classic reconstructions are used with a final averaging of the image-based motion corrected gates

A positive property of the serial pipeline is the easy and straightforward implementation which is consequently not very error-prone. But since all dual gates need to be actually reconstructed, the fineness of the subdivision due to the dual gating is limited in practice (i.e., m and n need to be chosen rather small) as the noise level for the images used for registration is increased. This in turn results in a reduced compensation of the motion induced artifacts.

It should also be noted that the final averaging step could be replaced by a Motion Compensated Image Reconstruction (MCIR), as described in Sect. 3.2.3. An MCIR might lead to a better image quality [4, 80, 110] of the final image, however, at the cost of increased run-time.

3.2.2 Simplified Pipeline

The serial pipeline in Sect. 3.2.1 requires many registration steps operating on the individual noisy dual gates. We propose a *simplified pipeline* for cardiac PET motion correction based on our previous work in [119] to reduce the $m \cdot n - 1$ motion estimation steps which are necessary in the serial approach. The main idea of the simplified pipeline is to decouple respiratory and cardiac motion estimation. Instead of matching all $m \cdot n - 1$ gates to an assigned reference gate, only $m - 1$ respiratory matching steps with subsequent $n - 1$ cardiac matching steps are performed.

It is assumed that respiratory and cardiac motion are independent to a certain degree. This allows the independent, respectively successive, estimation of respiratory and cardiac motion. The transformation for a specific dual gate T_i^j (respiratory phase $i \in \{1, \ldots, m\}$ and cardiac phase $j \in \{1, \ldots, n\}$) with respect to the reference gate $\mathcal{R}$ is determined by concatenating the corresponding respiratory ($\mathbf{y}_i$) and cardiac ($\mathbf{y}^j$) transformation, i.e., $\mathcal{R} \approx \mathcal{M}^{\mathrm{MP}}(T_i^j, \mathbf{y}_i \circ \mathbf{y}^j)$ using the mass-preserving transformation model $\mathcal{M}^{\mathrm{MP}}$ from Definition 2.11. Thereby $\mathbf{y}_i$ (respectively $\mathbf{y}^j$) denotes the transformation for the respiratory phase i (cardiac phase j) with respect to the respiratory (cardiac) phase of the reference gate. Consequently, $\mathbf{y}_i$ ($\mathbf{y}^j$) is the identity if i (j) represents the respiratory (cardiac) reference gate number. The simplified pipeline is illustrated in Fig. 3.2 and consists of the following steps:

1. Determination of the dual gating signal
2. Reconstruction of all dual gates   ($m \cdot n$ resulting images)
3. Averaging of all cardiac phases for each respiratory gate   (m resulting images)
4. Respiratory motion estimation   ($m - 1$ registration tasks)
5. Averaging of all motion corrected respiratory phases
   for each cardiac gate   (n resulting images)
6. Cardiac motion estimation   ($n - 1$ registration tasks)
7. Averaging of all motion corrected dual gates   (1 resulting image)

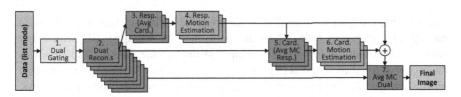

Fig. 3.2 Schematic illustration of the simplified pipeline [119]. The dual motion is decomposed into its respiratory and cardiac component. Classic reconstructions are used with a final averaging of the image-based motion corrected gates

Motion due to respiration is almost rigid for the region of the heart in contrast to the highly non-linear cardiac motion. It is therefore advisable to first estimate and eliminate the respiratory and subsequently the cardiac motion component. Given this order of the correction steps, we will discuss the individual steps in more detail in the following.

For respiratory motion estimation, a naive strategy could be the selection of all respiratory images from the whole set of dual gates belonging to only one single cardiac phase (from one column of the matrix of dual gates). However, the robustness of the motion estimation process can be increased by averaging all cardiac gates for each respiratory phase (step 3) which results in an improved SNR (averaging of all columns in the matrix of dual gates). Consequently, the resulting respiratory gated images are still blurred due to motion induced by the cardiac cycle. Nevertheless, this should only weakly affect the estimation of the locally almost rigid respiratory motion.

The cardiac gates (step 5) are obtained by applying the already estimated respiratory motion to each dual gate, according to its respiratory gate affiliation, and by performing an averaging of all respiratory gates for each cardiac phase. The resulting images represent cardiac gates which are already corrected for respiratory motion and are thus well suited for cardiac motion estimation.

The uncoupling of respiratory and cardiac motion estimation allows for a motion dependent parameter settings by incorporating prior knowledge. No large volume changes are to be expected during respiratory motion estimation resulting in a strong penalization of the volume term in hyperelastic regularization, cf. Definition 2.7. In contrast, one might want to allow volume changes to a certain degree in cardiac motion estimation due to the strong non-linear behavior, which can be considered by a weaker penalization of the volume term.

The total processing time of the simplified pipeline will be decreased compared to the serial pipeline as the total number of registration tasks is reduced from $m \times n - 1$ to $m + n - 2$. As for the serial pipeline, the averaging steps could also be replaced by MCIRs which is the main motivation of the modified pipeline described in the next section.

3.2.3   Simplified Pipeline with MCIRs

The advantage of the simplified pipeline over the serial pipeline is the reduced number of registration tasks which are performed on averaged data with better statistics. This reduces the overall registration time of the pipeline and stabilizes the motion estimation in terms of robustness against noise. We propose a *simplified pipeline* with *Motion Compensated Image Reconstructions* (MCIRs) which allows, in addition to the above mentioned advantages, a fine dual gating. In addition, MCIRs feature an improved image quality compared to the averaging approach [4, 80, 110].

For pure respiratory motion correction an optimal number of 8–10 gates was found [36]. Due to the high non-linearity of cardiac motion, the number of cardiac gates in pure cardiac gating should be chosen at least as high as the number of respiratory gates to finely resolve the complex motion. Transferring this directly to dual gating, a 10×10 matrix of 100 dual gates with highly reduced motion and, more importantly, highly reduced statistics per gate would result. In the previously described approaches (serial pipeline and simplified pipeline) a rather low number of gates was used (5×5 gating in [51, 119]) as the actual reconstruction of all 100 gates would have lead to too high noise levels. To overcome this limitation, the simplified pipeline is extended in this section by using MCIRs instead of averaging of images. The idea of MCIR is to include the motion into the reconstruction process [80] instead of applying it sequentially to the already reconstructed images. This allows a finer dual gating as the actual reconstruction of all individual $m \times n$ gates is no longer required. Instead, only m respiratory and n cardiac gates need to be reconstructed (plus the final reconstruction) where each actually reconstructed image contains a higher SNR compared to a single gate. The simplified pipeline with MCIRs is illustrated in Fig. 3.3 and consists of the following steps:

1. Determination of the dual gating signal
2. Reconstruction of all respiratory gates   (m resulting images)
3. Respiratory motion estimation   ($m - 1$ registration tasks)
4. Respiratory MCIR of all cardiac gates   (n resulting images)
5. Cardiac motion estimation   ($n - 1$ registration tasks)
6. Respiratory and cardiac MCIR   (1 resulting image)

The cardiac gates in step 4 are reconstructed based on the respiratory motion information gained in step 3. Instead of an image-based respiratory motion correction of each gate with a subsequent averaging of all respiratory phases for each cardiac gate, respiratory motion is applied during respiratory motion compensated reconstructions.

All available image information is put into one big respiratory and cardiac MCIR in step 6. The transformation for a specific dual gate is determined by concatenating the corresponding respiratory and cardiac transformation from steps 3 and 5 as described in the previous section for the simplified pipeline.

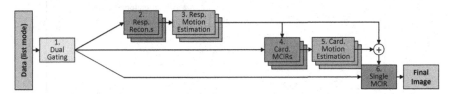

Fig. 3.3 Schematic illustration of the simplified pipeline with MCIRs [54]. The classic reconstructions of the simplified pipeline are replaced by MCIRs. The reconstruction of all single dual gates is no longer necessary

The total number of reconstructions of the simplified pipeline with MCIRs is $m + n + 1$ compared to $m \cdot n$ reconstructions for the serial and pure simplified pipeline. As the computational complexity of MCIR is higher compared to classic reconstructions this results in a reduction of produced images but not automatically in a simultaneous reduction of the total reconstruction time of the pipeline. Empirically, it has been found that both approaches have a comparable total run-time behavior.

Table 3.1 Comparison of the serial and the simplified pipeline with MCIRs. The numbers for $e(\boldsymbol{y},\boldsymbol{y}_{GT})$ and NCC are average values over all 25 dual gates. The range of the Jacobian map represents the global minimum and maximum for all images. The maximum endpoint error is also the global maximum error for all images

	Serial pipeline	Simplified pipeline w/MCIRs
$e(\boldsymbol{y},\boldsymbol{y}_{GT})$	1.60 mm	1.50 mm
$e^{\max}(\boldsymbol{y},\boldsymbol{y}_{GT})$	8.20 mm	8.19 mm
$\min_{\boldsymbol{x}}\{\det(\nabla\boldsymbol{y}(\boldsymbol{x}))\}$	0.65	0.64
$\max_{\boldsymbol{x}}\{\det(\nabla\boldsymbol{y}(\boldsymbol{x}))\}$	1.18	1.19
$\mathrm{NCC}(\mathcal{T},\mathcal{R})$	0.61	0.61
$\mathrm{NCC}(\mathcal{M}^{\mathrm{MP}}(\mathcal{T},\boldsymbol{y}),\mathcal{R})$	0.88	0.87

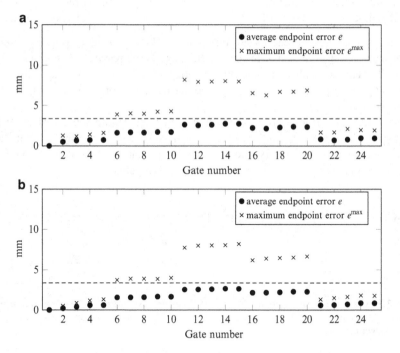

Fig. 3.4 Average endpoint error e and maximum endpoint error $e^{\max}$ are shown for each gate for the serial and the simplified pipeline with MCIRs. The voxel size of 3.375 mm is indicated by the *dashed horizontal line*. The five respiratory gates for the first cardiac gate are shown with the gate numbers 1–5. The five respiratory gates for the second cardiac gate are shown with the gate numbers 6–10, etc. (**a**) Serial pipeline. (**b**) Simplified pipeline with MCIRs

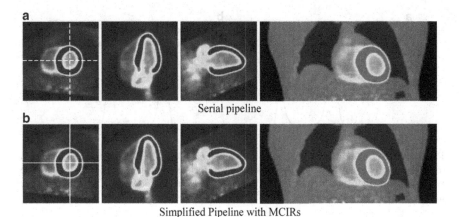

Fig. 3.5   The cardiac planes (SA, HLA, VLA) and a representative coronal plane of the final image are shown for the serial pipeline in (**a**) and for the simplified pipeline with MCIRs in (**b**). For the coronal slices the μ-map is overlaid with the respective PET data. Line profiles indicated in the SA views are given in Fig. 3.6

3.2.4   Results

The serial pipeline and the simplified pipeline with MCIRs are applied to the same XCAT software phantom data that is used for the evaluation part of Sect. 2.3. The underlying data is described in more detail in Sect. 2.1.6. To be precise, the SSD VAMPIRE result in Fig. 2.7 represents exactly the result of the simplified pipeline with MCIRs to be discussed in the following. We do not include the simplified pipeline (*without* MCIRs) into this evaluation as the strategy is very close to the strategy of the simplified pipeline *with* MCIRs and MCIRs are generally advantageous over simple averaging [4, 110].

The average values (over all 25 gates) of the validation criteria described in the evaluation part of Sect. 2.3 are summarized in Table 3.1 for both pipelines. The values for the average and maximum endpoint error are further plotted in Fig. 3.4 for each gate individually. For all gates the average endpoint errors are below the voxel size. The final corrected images of the two approaches are shown in Fig. 3.5. The images are essentially very similar which is supported by the line profiles in Fig. 3.6. On the one hand, this shows that we do not lose any accuracy due to the approximation of the decoupled respiratory and cardiac motion using the simplified pipeline. On the other hand, we are now able to apply our motion correction strategy to PET data with a fine dual gating. The improvement due to motion correction becomes obvious by comparing the results in Fig. 3.5 with Fig. 2.10b.

In conclusion, we have seen several methods for motion correction in gated PET. We discussed a pure gating-based technique with optimal gating. We further presented various methods combining gating with motion estimation and correction. For the particular case of dual gated PET the presented simplified pipelines provide

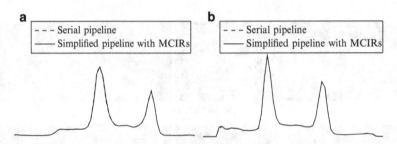

Fig. 3.6 Line profiles of the SA views in the left column of Fig. 3.5. The *dashed line* represents the serial pipeline and the *solid line* the simplified pipeline with MCIRs. The line profiles are very similar which is supported by the high similarity of the images in Fig. 3.5. (**a**) Line profiles x dimension. (**b**) Line profiles y dimension

a powerful tool. They provide a framework for fast (reduced number of registration tasks) and robust (high SNR of the images in each registration task) motion correction. The serial pipelines and the simplified pipeline with MCIRs show similar good results whereas the simplified pipeline with MCIRs has a lower average endpoint error in addition to a reduced number of registration and reconstruction tasks.

Chapter 4
Further Developments in PET Motion Correction

We have discussed methods for PET motion estimation and motion correction in the previous chapters. In particular, a priori knowledge about the image generation process, in terms of mass-preservation, was utilized to improve the motion estimates needed for the advanced correction pipelines. This chapter gives an outlook of potential improvements and modifications of the presented methods and future advances of PET motion correction in general. The proposed improvements of the process of motion estimation and motion correction are given by, e.g., extracting motion from accompanying MRI scans instead of the PET data itself. Further, we briefly discuss future developments of PET motion correction in clinical applications.

4.1 Future Work of VAMPIRE and MPOF

The methods described in Chaps. 2 and 3 describe the general proceeding for mass-preserving motion estimation and motion correction in PET. In the following, we discuss some potential improvements of the described proceeding. These modifications are:

- Using an improved gating technique,
- Extension to a spatial-temporal approach,
- Application to dynamic PET data.

Further improvements by parameter optimization is not discussed in great detail. We just provide the following list of starting points. It is desirable to determine the

- Optimal number of respiratory and cardiac gates (cf. Sect. 3.2.3),
- Optimal regularization parameters (cf. Sects. 2.1.2 and 2.2.3),

© The Author(s) 2015
F. Gigengack et al., *Motion Correction in Thoracic Positron Emission Tomography*,
SpringerBriefs in Electrical and Computer Engineering,
DOI 10.1007/978-3-319-08392-6_4

- Optimal spline control point spacing/number of spline control points (cf. Sect. 2.1.3), and the
- Influence of additional spline control points outside the image domain.

4.1.1 Gating

The gating schemes for VAMPIRE used in [51] and MPOF in [37] use an equidistant time-based gating for the cardiac cycle. A more sophisticated cardiac gating with time varying cardiac gates [127] or with grouping of cardiac phases [74] could better resolve the cardiac phases (in particular regarding the systole) and should be considered in future work.

For respiratory motion, the proposed amplitude-based gating has the advantage of (almost) equal statistics in each gate, which manifests itself in a comparable noise level in the reconstructed images. This allows us to choose a constant set of regularization parameters for all motion estimation tasks. The downside of this gating scheme is the varying motion blur in different gates. Infrequent motion states feature an increased blurring induced by motion. A phase-based gating scheme would allow to create gates with equal motion blur in each gate, however, with the effect of different SNRs in the gates. The optimal trade-off between remaining motion and statistics per gate should thus be explored. This is directly related to the analysis of the optimal number of dual gates, which is not addressed in this work but interesting to analyze, cf. [36].

4.1.2 Spatial-Temporal Approach

Respiratory and cardiac motion is cyclic and smooth over time. It should thus be taken advantage of this information. The approaches described in Chap. 2 estimate the motion between each motion phase and the reference phase independently. Modifications could be an estimation of motion between each phase and its subsequent phase to keep the expected motion vectors small [73]. This is particularly interesting for optical flow methods due to the Taylor linearization. Another extension is to explore the cyclic nature of motion [83]. As hyperelastic regularization allows for large motion, this is not essential in the case of VAMPIRE. Still, a global smoothness constraint which accounts for smooth transitions and cyclicality should be investigated to further improve the robustness of motion estimation towards noise.

Klein et al. [73] also propose a tissue-dependent regularization in their work by modeling the incompressibility of myocardial tissue. If different tissue compartment are given, e.g., by applying a prior segmentation, non-uniform regularization could be applied to incorporate further a priori knowledge about tissue-dependent motion behavior.

4.1.3 Dynamic PET

The applications of motion estimation and correction discussed in this book assume that the tracer is already accumulated in the tissue. We expect no considerable tracer dynamics between different motion phases. However, dynamic PET scans are also acquired in daily clinical routine and should thus also be corrected for motion. Consequently, simultaneous estimation of tracer kinetics and motion in dynamic PET scans is an important and interesting field of application.

Motion estimation in dynamic PET brings up some challenges, which are presumably the reason why motion correction in dynamic PET is more or less neglected so far. We have already seen that the main assumption of most motion estimation techniques is that corresponding points in different images have approximately the same intensity. In the case of dynamic PET we cannot expect similar intensities at corresponding points as the uptake of radioactivity varies for each individual organ over time according to the tracer dynamics. As in the case of mass-preservation, this deviation from the assumption of similar intensities needs to be modeled explicitly. We thus have to model the tracer dynamics, e.g., using kinetic modeling [26, 120], in addition to the motion estimation. A possible sequential correction scheme could be:

1. Respiratory gating using the whole data set (tracer dynamics are averaged out).
2. Estimation of respiratory motion (with mass-preservation).
3. Kinetic modeling using the whole data set (respiratory motion corrected).
4. Cardiac gating of the whole data set (respiratory motion corrected and compensated for tracer dynamics).
5. Estimation of cardiac motion (with mass-preservation).
6. Reconstruction of the final image which is corrected for respiratory and cardiac motion and tracer dynamics.

A joint (simultaneous) estimation of motion and tracer dynamics would also be interesting. Motion and tracer dynamics could be estimated using a joint functional with an alternating optimization.

4.2 Recent Developments in Gating

With the aim of an improved image quality of the desired final motion corrected image, the data basis for motion estimation can also be attacked. In our case the data basis is given by the output of the preceding gating procedure. A data-driven gating technique called *gating+* is proposed by Kesner et al. in [70]. The method operates in the frequency domain and aims to resolve motion while preserving the high SNR of the ungated image. An adaptive band-pass filter is applied in frequency space to each voxel individually. The cut-off frequency is chosen as the frequency where the signal of the analyzed voxel of the current gate starts to match the signal of a randomly gated image. The randomly gated image is created based on random (motion independent) trigger signals and represents thus the random noise.

Another approach for an improvement of the gated images is presented in [24] by Büther et al. The idea is to attach external markers to the patient to guarantee a sufficiently strong signal which can be used by their data-driven gating technique. Consequently, the proposed method is also applicable to patients with low global uptake.

4.3 Influence of Motion on PET Attenuation Correction

In oncological PET imaging, using CT or MRI to generate PET attenuation maps, respiratory motion may introduce artifacts at the position of the diaphragm due to μ values derived from incorrect respiratory phases. Therefore, there is a specific need to solve this registration problem in hybrid PET imaging. No matter whether gating or reconstruction-based correction methods are being used, the respiratory phase at which a corresponding CT or MRI images has been acquired needs to be known accurately. Apart from various techniques for predicting the respiratory phase, such as intrinsic or extrinsic markers, navigators, etc., there has been another elegant way of generating μ-maps for proper attenuation correction. With the advent of Time-Of-Flight (TOF)-PET in clinical PET/CT scanners, an old idea [103] of jointly reconstructing emission and transmission data within an integrated iterative reconstruction algorithm became reality, called Maximum Likelihood reconstruction of Attenuation and Activity (MLAA) [62,113]. Using this approach, a μ-map is reconstructed that is, by definition, registered to the corresponding emission image obviating the need for additional attenuation estimations. In addition, truncation problems of CT and MRI may be solved with this approach leading to more accurate and quantitative PET images [102].

4.4 Future Advances Using PET/MRI

One big issue in PET-based motion correction is the relatively low information content in the PET images. Motion can only be estimated in regions of sufficiently high tracer uptake which may limit intrinsic motion estimation approaches. A global motion estimation and correction is thus hardly achievable. The clinically relevant structures are usually given by these high uptake regions, which makes PET-based motion correction practicable in many applications. However, small lesions might be invisible in the uncorrected PET image due to motion blurring and reliable estimation of motion is hardly possible. As such lesions are of great clinical relevance, the idea is to make them visible again by deriving motion fields from auxiliary measurements. As mentioned in Sect. 1.5.1, the required motion information for PET motion correction can be estimated based on MRI images in the case of a simultaneous PET/MRI scan. The advantage of MRI-based motion estimation is that information is globally available and not only in areas of high molecular signals, as in the case of PET. In addition, MRI has a very high soft tissue contrast in comparison to CT imaging offering motion information in all parts of the thorax and abdomen.

Although MRI offers very fast image acquisition techniques for 2D imaging, high-resolution and fast 3D imaging is still challenging. For real-time respiratory gating for PET motion correction, respiratory sampling times of 400–700 ms may be fast enough to provide a good sampling of all respiratory phases, as has been shown recently [21,39,45,136]. For cardiac gating, higher sampling frequencies are mandatory in order to follow the heart motion in real-time. A further challenge is the subsequent spatial and temporal alignment of the PET and MRI data.

MRI-based motion correction of PET data is still under development, but already demonstrated its feasibility showing promising result. In [43] a joint registration functional is presented to make use of motion information derived from PET and MRI data simultaneously. The proposed method is demonstrated to achieve a lower local registration error and better recovery of lesion activity. Beyond the success of correction methods in PET/CT, MRI will have a major impact on motion correction strategies improving the quantitative accuracy of PET images. A more far-reaching discussion on this topic can be found in [114].

4.5 Motion Correction in Clinical Practice

Although many attempts were made to develop motion correction techniques in PET/CT, only a few methods found their way into clinical practice. Of those, cardiac and respiratory gating procedures are nowadays widely accepted but are associated with the disadvantage of an elongated scanning time. Only recently, amplitude-based respiratory gating has been introduced using internal or external devices for estimation the respiratory phase.

Gating procedures using PET list mode data to estimate respiratory motion show promising results and already provide effective methods for clinical motion correction. More clinical studies will have to prove whether these methods are robust enough for dedicated correction tasks. It is obvious that PET data driven techniques are only successful in cases, where sufficient contrast of PET uptake is present for the moving structures of interest. Moreover, motion estimation using PET data alone may only provide information at high contrast regions, underestimating motion at low contrast areas. Moving lesions with low contrast, however, should benefit mostly from motion correction techniques, since those lesions, that are not be detectable on static PET images, may become visible after motion correction.

In motion correction areas where PET-CT has clear disadvantages, whole-body simultaneous PET-MRI offers new elegant ways of accurate correction. The MRI-derived motion fields can be used directly in the PET reconstruction in a non-rigid motion correction approach. Thus, PET-MRI has the potential of completely removing motion effects without the loss of signal-to-noise ratio. At the same time, MRI provides useful additional clinical information [114].

Besides improvements in clinical diagnostics, motion estimation using PET-MRI may have another clinical impact on accurate radiotherapy treatment planning. Intensity-modulated radiotherapy and dose painting approaches have to take the respiratory motion into account during treatment. Here, PET-MRI provides not only quantitative molecular information about a lesion during treatment, but describes also the lesion's path during the respiratory cycle within the same imaging sessions.

Certainly, within the next decades PET-MRI will have an ever increasing importance with respect to accurate and quantitative PET imaging. More sophisticated non-rigid motion correction techniques will find their way into clinical practice and will improve the detectability and diagnostic accuracy of moving structures.

References

1. L. Armijo, Minimization of functions having Lipschitz continuous first partial derivatives. Pac. J. Math. **16**(1), 1–3 (1966)
2. V. Arsigny, O. Commowick, N. Ayache, X. Pennec, A fast and Log-Euclidean polyaffine framework for locally linear registration. J. Math. Imaging Vis. **33**(2), 222–238 (2009)
3. V. Arsigny, P. Fillard, X. Pennec, N. Ayache, Fast and simple calculus on tensors in the Log-Euclidean framework, in *Medical Image Computing and Computer-Assisted Intervention* (Springer, Berlin/Heidelberg, 2005), pp. 115–122
4. E. Asma, R. Manjeshwar, K. Thielemans, Theoretical comparison of motion correction techniques for PET image reconstruction, in *IEEE Nuclear Science Symposium and Medical Imaging Conference (NSS/MIC)*, San Diego, 2006, vol. 3, pp. 1762–1767
5. B.B. Avants, P.T. Schoenemann, J.C. Gee, Lagrangian frame diffeomorphic image registration: morphometric comparison of human and chimpanzee cortex. Med. Image Anal. **10**(3), 397–412 (2006)
6. W. Bai, M. Brady, Respiratory motion correction in PET images. Phys. Med. Biol. **54**, 2719–2736 (2009)
7. W. Bai, M. Brady, Spatio-temporal image registration for respiratory motion correction in PET, in *IEEE International Symposium on Biomedical Imaging: From Nano to Macro*, Boston, 2009, pp. 426–429
8. W. Bai, M. Brady, Motion correction and attenuation correction for respiratory gated PET images. IEEE Trans. Med. Imaging **30**(2), 351–365 (2011)
9. J.L. Barron, D.J. Fleet, S.S. Beauchemin, Performance of optical flow techniques. Int. J. Comput. Vis. **12**(1), 43–77 (1994)
10. D. Béréziat, I. Herlin, L. Younes, A generalized optical flow constraint and its physical interpretation, in *IEEE Conference on Computer Vision and Pattern Recognition*, Hilton Head, 2000, vol. 2, pp. 487–492
11. T. Beyer, G. Antoch, T. Blodgett, L.F. Freudenberg, T. Akhurst, S. Mueller, Dual-modality PET/CT imaging: the effect of respiratory motion on combined image quality in clinical oncology. Eur. J. Nucl. Med. Mol. Imaging **30**, 588–596 (2003)
12. M. Blume, *Joint Image and Motion Reconstruction for Positron Emission Tomography*. PhD thesis, Technische Universität München, 2011
13. M. Blume, A. Martinez-Möller, A. Keil, N. Navab, M. Rafecas, Joint reconstruction of image and motion in gated positron emission tomography. IEEE Trans. Med. Imaging **29**(11), 1892–1906 (2010)

14. M. Blume, N. Navab, M. Rafecas, Joint image and motion reconstruction for PET using a B-spline motion model. Phys. Med. Biol. **57**(24), 8249–8270 (2012)

15. F.A Bornemann, P. Deuflhard, The cascadic multigrid method for elliptic problems. Numer. Math. **75**(2), 135–152 (1996)

16. J. Brewer, Kronecker products and matrix calculus in system theory. IEEE Trans. Circuits Syst. **25**(9), 772–781 (1978)

17. C. Broit, *Optimal Registration of Deformed Images*. PhD thesis, University of Pennsylvania, Philadelphia, 1981

18. L.G. Brown, A survey of image registration techniques. ACM Comput. Surv. **24**(4), 325–376 (1992)

19. A. Bruhn, J. Weickert, C. Schnörr, Lucas/Kanade meets Horn/Schunck: combining local and global optic flow methods. Int. J. Comput. Vis. **61**, 211–231 (2005)

20. C. Brune, *4D Imaging in Tomography and Optical Nanoscopy*. PhD thesis, University of Münster, 2010

21. C. Buerger, C. Tsoumpas, A. Aitken, A.P. King, P. Schleyer, V. Schulz, P.K. Marsden, T. Schaeffter, Investigation of MR-based attenuation correction and motion compensation for hybrid PET/MR. IEEE Trans. Nucl. Sci. **59**(5), 1967–1976 (2012)

22. M. Burger, J. Modersitzki, L. Ruthotto, A hyperelastic regularization energy for image registration. SIAM J. Sci. Comput. **35**(1), B132–B148 (2013)

23. F. Büther, M. Dawood, L. Stegger, F. Wübbeling, M. Schäfers, O. Schober, K.P. Schäfers, List mode-driven cardiac and respiratory gating in PET. J. Nucl. Med. **50**(5), 674–681 (2009)

24. F. Büther, I. Ernst, J. Hamill, H.T. Eich, O. Schober, M. Schäfers, K.P. Schäfers, External radioactive markers for pet data-driven respiratory gating in positron emission tomography. Eur. J. Nucl. Med. Mol. Imaging **40**(4), 602–614 (2013)

25. Cardiac planes, http://www.nuclearcardiologyseminars.net/images/cardiacplanes1.gif. Online; Accessed 06 Apr 2014

26. R.E. Carson, Tracer kinetic modeling in PET, in *Positron Emission Tomography: Basic Sciences* (Springer, New York, 2005), pp. 127–159

27. H. Chang, J.M. Fitzpatrick, A technique for accurate magnetic resonance imaging in the presence of field inhomogeneities. IEEE Trans. Med. Imaging **11**(3), 319–329 (1992)

28. P. Charbonnier, L. Blanc-Feraud, G. Aubert, M. Barlaud, Two deterministic half-quadratic regularization algorithms for computed imaging, in *IEEE International Conference on Image Processing*, Austin, 1994, vol. 2, pp. 168–172

29. S.Y. Chun, T.G. Reese, J. Ouyang, B. Guerin, C. Catana, X. Zhu, N.M. Alpert, G. El Fakhri, MRI-based nonrigid motion correction in simultaneous PET/MRI. J. Nucl. Med. **53**(8), 1284–1291 (2012)

30. P.G. Ciarlet, *Mathematical Elasticity: Three-Dimensional Elasticity* (North Holland, Amsterdam/New York, 1988)

31. T. Corpetti, É. Mémin, P. Pérez, Dense motion analysis in fluid imagery, in *European Conference on Computer Vision*, Copenhagen (Springer, 2002), pp. 676–691

32. M. Dawood, *Respiratory Motion Correction on 3D Positron Emission Tomography Images*. PhD thesis, University of Münster, 2008

33. M. Dawood, C. Brune, F. Büther, X. Jiang, M. Burger, O. Schober, M. Schäfers, K.P. Schäfers, A continuity equation based optical flow method for cardiac motion correction in 3D PET data, in *Medical Image Computing and Computer-Assisted Intervention*, vol. 6326 (Springer, Berlin/Heidelberg, 2010), pp. 88–97

34. M. Dawood, F. Büther, X. Jiang, K.P. Schäfers, Respiratory motion correction in 3-D PET data with advanced optical flow algorithms. IEEE Trans. Med. Imaging **27**(8), 1164–1175 (2008)

35. M. Dawood, F. Büther, N. Lang, O. Schober, K.P. Schäfers, Respiratory gating in positron emission tomography: a quantitative comparison of different gating schemes. Med. Phys. **34**(7), 3067–3076 (2007)

36. M. Dawood, F. Büther, L. Stegger, X. Jiang, O. Schober, M. Schäfers, K.P. Schäfers, Optimal number of respiratory gates in positron emission tomography: a cardiac patient study. Med. Phys. **36**(5), 1775–1784 (2009)

37. M. Dawood, F. Gigengack, X. Jiang, K.P. Schäfers, A mass conservation-based optical flow method for cardiac motion correction in 3D-PET. Med. Phys. **40**(1), 012505 (2013)

38. M. Dawood, X. Jiang, K. Schäfers (eds.), *Correction Techniques in Emission Tomography*. Series in Medical Physics and Biomedical Engineering (CRC, Boca Raton, 2012)

39. N. Dikaios, D. Izquierdo-Garcia, M.J. Graves, V. Mani, Z.A. Fayad, T.D. Fryer, MRI-based motion correction of thoracic PET: initial comparison of acquisition protocols and correction strategies suitable for simultaneous PET/MRI systems. Eur. Radiol. **22**(2), 439–446 (2012)

40. M. Droske, M. Rumpf, A variational approach to nonrigid morphological image registration. SIAM J. Appl. Math. **64**(2), 668–687 (2003)

41. Y.E. Erdi, S.A. Nehmeh, T. Mulnix, J.L. Humm, C.C. Watson, PET performance measurements for an LSO-based combined PET/CT scanner using the national electrical manufacturers association NU 2-2001 standard. J. Nucl. Med. **45**(5), 813–821 (2004)

42. Y.E. Erdi, S.A. Nehmeh, T. Pan, A. Pevsner, K.E. Rosenzweig, G. Mageras, E.D. Yorke, H. Schoder, W. Hsiao, O.D. Squire, P. Vernon, J.B. Ashman, H. Mostafavi, S.M. Larson, J.L. Humm, The CT motion quantitation of lung lesions and its impact on PET-measured SUVs. J. Nucl. Med. **45**(8), 1287–1292 (2004)

43. M. Fieseler, F. Gigengack, X. Jiang, K.P. Schäfers, Motion correction of whole-body PET data with a joint PET-MRI registration functional. BioMed. Eng. Online **13**(Suppl 1), S2 (2014)

44. M. Fieseler, T. Kosters, F. Gigengack, H. Braun, H.H. Quick, K.P. Schäfers, X. Jiang, Motion correction in PET-MRI: a human torso phantom study, in *IEEE Nuclear Science Symposium and Medical Imaging Conference (NSS/MIC)*, Valencia, 2011, pp. 3586–3588

45. M. Fieseler, H. Kugel, F. Gigengack, T. Kösters, F. Büther, H.H. Quick, C. Faber, X. Jiang, K.P. Schäfers, A dynamic thorax phantom for the assessment of cardiac and respiratory motion correction in PET/MRI: a preliminary evaluation. Nucl. Instrum. Methods Phys. Res. Sect. A: Accel. Spectrom. Detect. Assoc. Equip. **702**, 59–63 (2013)

46. L. Fin, P. Bailly, J. Daouk, M.-E. Meyer, Motion correction based on an appropriate system matrix for statistical reconstruction of respiratory-correlated PET acquisitions. Comput. Methods Programs Biomed. **96**(3), e1–e9 (2009)

47. B. Fischer, J. Modersitzki, Fast diffusion registration. AMS Contemp. Math. Inverse Probl. Image Anal. Med. Imaging **313**, 117–129 (2002)

48. B. Fischer, J. Modersitzki, Ill-posed medicine—an introduction to image registration. Inverse Probl. **24**, 034008 (2008)

49. F. Gigengack, M. Fieseler, D. Tenbrinck, X. Jiang, Image processing techniques in emission tomography, in *Correction Techniques in Emission Tomography*. Series in Medical Physics and Biomedical Engineering (Taylor & Francis, London, 2012), pp. 119–156

50. F. Gigengack, L. Ruthotto, M. Burger, C.H. Wolters, X. Jiang, K.P. Schäfers, Motion correction of cardiac PET using mass-preserving registration, in *IEEE Nuclear Science Symposium and Medical Imaging Conference (NSS/MIC)*, Knoxville, 2010, pp. 3317–3319

51. F. Gigengack, L. Ruthotto, M. Burger, C.H. Wolters, X. Jiang, K.P. Schäfers, Motion correction in dual gated cardiac PET using mass-preserving image registration. IEEE Trans. Med. Imaging **31**(3), 698–712 (2012)

52. F. Gigengack, L. Ruthotto, X. Jiang, M. Burger, J. Modersitzki, C.H. Wolters, K.P. Schäfers, VAMPIRE, http://vampire.uni-muenster.de

53. F. Gigengack, L. Ruthotto, X. Jiang, J. Modersitzki, M. Burger, S. Hermann, K.P. Schäfers, Atlas-based whole-body PET-CT segmentation using a passive contour distance, in *Proceedings of MICCAI Workshop on Medical Computer Vision*, Nice (Springer, 2012), pp. 82–92

54. F. Gigengack, L. Ruthotto, T. Kösters, X. Jiang, J. Modersitzki, M. Burger, C.H. Wolters, K.P. Schäfers, Pipeline for motion correction in dual gated PET, in *IEEE Nuclear Science Symposium and Medical Imaging Conference (NSS/MIC)*, Anaheim, 2012

55. P.E. Gill, W. Murray, M.H. Wright, *Practical Optimization* (Academic, London, 1981)

56. G.W. Goerres, C. Burger, E. Kamel, B. Seifert, A.H. Kaim, A. Buck, T.C. Buehler, G.K. von Schulthess, Respiration-induced attenuation artifact at PET/CT: technical considerations. Radiology **226**(3), 906–910 (2003)

57. V. Gorbunova, J. Sporring, P. Lo, M. Loeve, H.A. Tiddens, M. Nielsen, A. Dirksen, M. de Bruijne, Mass preserving image registration for lung CT. Med. Image Anal. **16**, 786–795 (2012)

58. B. Guérin, S. Cho, S.Y. Chun, X. Zhu, N.M. Alpert, G. El Fakhri, T. Reese, C Catana, Nonrigid PET motion compensation in the lower abdomen using simultaneous tagged-MRI and PET imaging. Med. Phys. **38**, 3025 (2011)

59. E. Haber, J. Modersitzki, Numerical methods for volume preserving image registration. Inverse Probl. **20**, 1621–1638 (2004)

60. E. Haber, J. Modersitzki, Image registration with guaranteed displacement regularity. Int. J. Comput. Vis. **71**(3), 361–372 (2007)

61. J. Hadamard, *Lectures on Cauchy's Problem in Linear Partial Differential Equations* (Yale University Press, New Haven, 1923)

62. J.J. Hamill, V.Y. Panin, TOF-MLAA for attenuation correction in thoracic PET/CT, in *IEEE Nuclear Science Symposium and Medical Imaging Conference (NSS/MIC)*, Anaheim, 2012, pp. 4040–4047

63. M. Holden, A review of geometric transformations for nonrigid body registration. IEEE Trans. Med. Imaging **27**(1), 111–128 (2008)

64. B.K.P. Horn, B.G. Schunck, Determining optical flow. Artif. Intell. **17**(1–3), 185–203 (1981)

65. H.M. Hudson, R.S. Larkin, Accelerated image reconstruction using ordered subsets of projection data. IEEE Trans. Med. Imaging **13**(4), 601–609 (1994)

66. B.F. Hutton, M. Braun, L. Thurfjell, D.Y. Lau, Image registration: an essential tool for nuclear medicine. Eur. J. Nucl. Med. **29**(4), 559–577 (2002)

67. D. Ionascu, S.B. Jiang, S. Nishioka, H. Shirato, R.I. Berbeco, Internal-external correlation investigations of respiratory induced motion of lung tumors. Med. Phys. **34**(10), 3893–903 (2007)

68. M.W. Jacobson, J.A. Fessler, Joint estimation of image and deformation parameters in motion-corrected PET, in *IEEE Nuclear Science Symposium and Medical Imaging Conference (NSS/MIC)*, Portland, 2003, vol. 5, pp. 3290–3294

69. S. Jan, G. Santin, D. Strul, S. Staelens, K. Assié, D. Autret, S. Avner, R. Barbier, M. Bardiès, P.M. Bloomfield, D. Brasse, V. Breton, P. Bruyndonckx, I. Buvat, A.F. Chatziioannou, Y. Choi, Y.H. Chung, C. Comtat, D. Donnarieix, L. Ferrer, S.J. Glick, C.J. Groiselle, D. Guez, P.-F. Honore, S. Kerhoas-Cavata, A.S. Kirov, V. Kohli, M. Koole, M. Krieguer, D.J. van der Laan, F. Lamare, G. Largeron, C. Lartizien, D. Lazaro, M.C. Maas, L. Maigne, F. Mayet, F. Melot, C. Merheb, E. Pennacchio, J. Perez, U. Pietrzyk, F.R. Rannou, M. Rey, D.R. Schaart, C.R. Schmidtlein, L. Simon, T.Y. Song, J.-M. Vieira, D. Visvikis, R. Van de Walle, E. Wieërs, C. Morel, GATE: a simulation toolkit for PET and SPECT. Phys. Med. Biol. **49**(19), 4543–4561 (2004)

70. A.L. Kesner, G. Abourbeh, E. Mishani, R. Chisin, S. Tshori, N. Freedman, Gating, enhanced gating, and beyond: information utilization strategies for motion management, applied to preclinical PET. EJNMMI Res. **3**(1), 29 (2013)

71. G.J. Klein, Forward deformation of PET volumes using material constraints, in *IEEE Workshop on Biomedical Image Analysis*, Santa Barbara, 1998, pp. 64–71

72. G.J. Klein, Forward deformation of PET volumes using non-uniform elastic material constraints, in *Information Processing in Medical Imaging* (Springer, New York, 1999), pp. 358–363

73. J.K. Klein, R.H. Huesman, Four dimensional processing of deformable cardiac PET data. Med. Image Anal. **6**(1), 29–46 (2002)

74. G.J. Klein, B.W. Reutter, M.H. Ho, J.H. Reed, R.H. Huesman, Real-time system for respiratory-cardiac gating in positron tomography. IEEE Trans. Nucl. Sci. **45**(4), 2139–2143 (1998)

75. G.J. Klein, B.W. Reutter, R.H. Huesman, Non-rigid summing of gated PET via optical flow, in *IEEE Nuclear Science Symposium and Medical Imaging Conference (NSS/MIC)*, Anaheim, 1996, vol. 2

76. T. Kokki, H. Sipilä, M. Teräs, T. Noponen, N. Durand-Schaefer, R. Klén, J. Knuuti, Dual gated PET/CT imaging of small targets of the heart: method description and testing with a dynamic heart phantom. J. Nucl. Cardiol. **17**, 71–84 (2009)

77. T. Kösters, K.P. Schäfers, F. Wübbeling, EMRECON, http://emrecon.uni-muenster.de

78. T. Kösters, K.P. Schäfers, F. Wübbeling, EMRECON: an expectation maximization based image reconstruction framework for emission tomography data, in *IEEE Nuclear Science Symposium and Medical Imaging Conference (NSS/MIC)*, Valencia, 2011

79. F. Lamare, T. Cresson, J. Savean, C. Cheze Le Rest, A.J. Reader, D. Visvikis, Respiratory motion correction for PET oncology applications using affine transformation of list mode data. Phys. Med. Biol. **52**(1), 121–140 (2007)

80. F. Lamare, M.J. Ledesma Carbayo, T. Cresson, G. Kontaxakis, A. Santos, C.C. Le Rest, A.J. Reader, D. Visvikis, List-mode-based reconstruction for respiratory motion correction in PET using non-rigid body transformations. Phys. Med. Biol. **52**(17), 5187–5204 (2007)

81. F. Lamare, M. Teras, T. Kokki, H. Fayad, O. Rimoldi, P.G. Camici, J. Knuuti, D. Visvikis, Correction of respiratory motion in dual gated cardiac imaging in PET/CT, in *IEEE Nuclear Science Symposium and Medical Imaging Conference (NSS/MIC)*, Dresden, 2008, pp. 5264–5269

82. N. Lang, M. Dawood, F. Büther, O. Schober, M. Schäfers, K.P. Schäfers, Organ movement reduction in PET/CT using dual-gated list-mode acquisition. Z. Med. Phys. **16**(1), 93–100 (2006)

83. L. Li, Y. Yang, Optical flow estimation for a periodic image sequence. IEEE Trans. Image Process. **19**(1), 1–10 (2010)

84. T. Li, B. Thorndyke, E. Schreibmann, Y. Yang, L. Xing, Model-based image reconstruction for four-dimensional PET. Med. Phys. **33**(5), 1288–1298 (2006)

85. D.C. Liu, J. Nocedal, On the limited memory BFGS method for large scale optimization. Math. Program. **45**, 503–528 (1989)

86. B.D. Lucas, T. Kanade, An iterative image registration technique with an application to stereo vision, in *Proceedings of 7th International Joint Conference on Artificial Intelligence*, Vancouver, 1981, pp. 674–679

87. G. Lucignani, Respiratory and cardiac motion correction with 4D PET imaging: shooting at moving targets. Eur. J. Nucl. Med. Mol. Imaging **36**(2), 315–319 (2009)

88. J.B. Maintz, M.A. Viergever, A survey of medical image registration. Med. Image Anal. **2**(1), 1–36 (1998)

89. B.A. Mair, D.R. Gilland, J. Sun, Estimation of images and nonrigid deformations in gated emission CT. IEEE Trans. Med. Imaging **25**(9), 1130–1144 (2006)

90. T. Mäkelä, P. Clarysse, O. Sipilä, N. Pauna, Q.C. Pham, T. Katila, I.E. Magnin, A review of cardiac image registration methods. IEEE Trans. Med. Imaging **21**(9), 1011–1021 (2002)

91. T. Marin, J.G. Brankov, Deformable left-ventricle mesh model for motion-compensated filtering in cardiac gated SPECT. Med. Phys. **37**(10), 5471–5481 (2010)

92. A. Martinez-Möller, D. Zikic, R. Botnar, R. Bundschuh, W. Howe, S. Ziegler, N. Navab, M. Schwaiger, S. Nekolla, Dual cardiac–respiratory gated PET: implementation and results from a feasibility study. Eur. J. Nucl. Med. Mol. Imaging **34**, 1447–1454 (2007)

93. B. McCane, K. Novins, D. Crannitch, B. Galvin, On benchmarking optical flow. Comput. Vis. Image Underst. **84**(1), 126–143 (2001)

94. J. Modersitzki, *Numerical Methods for Image Registration* (Oxford University Press, New York, 2004)

95. J. Modersitzki, *FAIR: Flexible Algorithms for Image Registration* (SIAM, Philadelphia, 2009)

96. Y. Nakamoto, B.B. Chin, C. Cohade, M. Osman, M. Tatsumi, R.L. Wahl, PET/CT: artifacts caused by bowel motion. Nucl. Med. Commun. **25**(3), 221–225 (2004)

97. R. Narayanan, J.A. Fessler, H. Park, C.R. Meyer, Diffeomorphic nonlinear transformations: a local parametric approach for image registration, in *Information Processing in Medical Imaging* (Springer, New York, 2005), pp. 174–185

98. S.A. Nehmeh, Y.E. Erdi, Respiratory motion in positron emission tomography/computed tomography: a review. Clin. Occup. Environ. Med. **38**(3), 167–176 (2008)

99. A. Neumaier, Solving ill-conditioned and singular linear systems: a tutorial on regularization. SIAM Rev. **40**(3), 636–666 (1998)

100. J. Nocedal, S.J. Wright, *Numerical Optimization* (Springer, New York, 2000)

101. G. Noetscher, S.N. Makarov, N. Clow, Modeling accuracy and features of body-area networks with out-of-body antennas at 402 MHz. IEEE Antennas Propag. Mag. **53**(4), 118–143 (2011)

102. J. Nuyts, G. Bal, F. Kehren, M. Fenchel, C. Michel, C. Watson, Completion of a truncated attenuation image from the attenuated PET emission data. IEEE Trans. Med. Imaging **32**(2), 237–246 (2013)

103. J. Nuyts, P. Dupont, S. Stroobants, R. Benninck, L. Mortelmans, P. Suetens, Simultaneous maximum a posteriori reconstruction of attenuation and activity distributions from emission sinograms. IEEE Trans. Med. Imaging **18**(5), 393–403 (1999)

104. J. Olesch, L. Ruthotto, H. Kugel, S. Skare, B. Fischer, C.H. Wolters, A variational approach for the correction of field-inhomogeneities in EPI sequences, in *SPIE Medical Imaging Conference*, San Diego, 2010

105. M.M. Osman, C. Cohade, Y. Nakamoto, L.T. Marshall, J.P. Leal, R.L. Wahl, Clinically significant inaccurate localization of lesions with PET/CT: frequency in 300 patients. J. Nucl. Med. **44**(2), 240–243 (2003)

106. M.M. Osman, C. Cohade, Y. Nakamoto, R.L. Wahl, Respiratory motion artifacts on PET emission images obtained using CT attenuation correction on PET-CT. Eur. J. Nucl. Med. Mol. Imaging **30**, 603–606 (2003)

107. X. Pennec, R. Stefanescu, V. Arsigny, P. Fillard, N. Ayache, Riemannian elasticity: a statistical regularization framework for non-linear registration, in *Medical Image Computing and Computer-Assisted Intervention* (Springer, Berlin/Heidelberg, 2005), pp. 943–950

108. Y. Petibon, J. Ouyang, X. Zhu, C. Huang, T.G. Reese, S.Y. Chun, Q. Li, G. El Fakhri, Cardiac motion compensation and resolution modeling in simultaneous PET-MR: a cardiac lesion detection study. Phys. Med. Biol. **58**(7), 2085 (2013)

109. M. Phelps, *PET: Molecular Imaging and Its Biological Applications* (Springer, New York, 2004)

110. I. Polycarpou, C. Tsoumpas, P.K. Marsden, Analysis and comparison of two methods for motion correction in PET imaging. Med. Phys. **39**, 6474–6483 (2012)

111. F. Qiao, T. Pan, J.W. Clark Jr., O.R. Mawlawi, A motion-incorporated reconstruction method for gated PET studies. Phys. Med. Biol. **51**(15), 3769–3783 (2006)

112. M. Reyes, G. Malandain, P.M. Koulibaly, M.A. González-Ballester, J. Darcourt, Model-based respiratory motion compensation for emission tomography image reconstruction. Phys. Med. Biol. **52**(12), 3579–3600 (2007)

113. A. Rezaei, M. Defrise, G. Bal, C. Michel, M. Conti, C. Watson, J. Nuyts, Simultaneous reconstruction of activity and attenuation in time-of-flight PET. IEEE Trans. Med. Imaging **31**(12), 2224–2233 (2012)

114. C. Rischpler, S.G. Nekolla, I. Dregely, M. Schwaiger, Hybrid PET/MR imaging of the heart: potential, initial experiences, and future prospects. J. Nucl. Med. **54**(3), 402–415 (2013)

115. T. Rohlfing, Image similarity and tissue overlaps as surrogates for image registration accuracy: widely used but unreliable. IEEE Trans. Med. Imaging **31**(2), 153–163 (2012)

116. D. Ruan, J.A. Fessler, J.M. Balter, R.I. Berbeco, S. Nishioka, H. Shirato, Inference of hysteretic respiratory tumor motion from external surrogates: a state augmentation approach. Phys. Med. Biol. **53**(11), 2923 (2008)

117. D. Rueckert, P. Aljabar, R.A. Heckemann, J.V. Hajnal, A. Hammers, Diffeomorphic registration using B-splines, in *Medical Image Computing and Computer-Assisted Intervention*, ed. by R. Larsen, M. Nielsen, J. Sporring. Volume 4191 of LNCS (Springer, Berlin/Heidelberg, 2006), pp. 702–709

118. L. Ruthotto, *Mass-Preserving Registration of Medical Images*. German diploma thesis (Mathematics), Institute for Computational and Applied Mathematics, University of Münster, 2010

119. L. Ruthotto, F. Gigengack, M. Burger, C.H. Wolters, X. Jiang, K.P. Schäfers, J. Modersitzki, A simplified pipeline for motion correction in dual gated cardiac PET, in *Bildverarbeitung für die Medizin* (Springer, Berlin/Heidelberg, 2012), pp. 51–56

120. K.C. Schmidt, F.E. Turkheimer, Kinetic modeling in positron emission tomography. Q. J. Nucl. Med. **46**(1), 70–85 (2002)

121. H. Schumacher, J. Modersitzki, B. Fischer, Combined reconstruction and motion correction in SPECT imaging. IEEE Trans. Nucl. Sci. **56**, 73–80 (2009)

122. A.J. Schwarz, M.O. Leach, Implications of respiratory motion for the quantification of 2D MR spectroscopic imaging data in the abdomen. Phys. Med. Biol. **45**(8), 2105–2116 (2000)

123. W.P. Segars, M. Mahesh, T.J. Beck, E.C. Frey, B.M.W. Tsui, Realistic CT simulation using the 4d XCAT phantom. Med. Phys. **35**(8), 3800–3808 (2008)

124. L.A. Shepp, Y. Vardi, Maximum likelihood reconstruction for emission tomography. IEEE Trans. Med. Imaging **1**(2), 113–122 (1982)

125. D. Sun, S. Roth, M.J. Black. A quantitative analysis of current practices in optical flow estimation and the principles behind them. Int. J. Comput. Vis. **106**(2), 115–137 (2014)

126. D. Tenbrinck, S. Schmid, X. Jiang, K.P. Schäfers, J. Stypmann, Histogram-based optical flow for motion estimation in ultrasound imaging. J. Math. Imaging Vis. **47**(1–2), 138–150 (2013)

127. M. Teräs, T. Kokki, N. Durand-Schaefer, T. Noponen, M. Pietilä, J. Kiss, E. Hoppela, H. Sipilä, J. Knuuti, Dual-gated cardiac PET–clinical feasibility study. Eur. J. Nucl. Med. Mol. Imaging **37**, 505–516 (2010)

128. K. Thielemans, E. Asma, R.M. Manjeshwar, Mass-preserving image registration using free-form deformation fields, in *IEEE Nuclear Science Symposium and Medical Imaging Conference (NSS/MIC)*, Orlando, 2009

129. H. Ue, H. Haneishi, H. Iwanaga, K. Suga, Nonlinear motion correction of respiratory-gated lung SPECT images. IEEE Trans. Med. Imaging **25**(4), 486–495 (2006)

130. A. Van Der Gucht, B. Serrano, F. Hugonnet, B. Paulmier, N. Garnier, M. Faraggi, Impact of a new respiratory amplitude-based gating technique in evaluation of upper abdominal PET lesions. Eur. J. Radiol. **83**(3), 509–515 (2014)

131. W. van Elmpt, J. Hamill, J. Jones, D. De Ruysscher, P. Lambin, M. Öllers, Optimal gating compared to 3D and 4D PET reconstruction for characterization of lung tumours. Eur. J. Nucl. Med. Mol. Imaging **38**, 843–855 (2011)

132. T. Vercauteren, X. Pennec, A. Perchant, N. Ayache, Diffeomorphic demons: efficient non-parametric image registration. NeuroImage **45**(1), S61–S72 (2009)

133. D. Visvikis, O. Barret, T.D. Fryer, A. Lamare, A. Turzo, Y. Bizais, C.C. Le Rest, Evaluation of respiratory motion effects in comparison with other parameters affecting PET image quality, in *IEEE Nuclear Science Symposium and Medical Imaging Conference (NSS/MIC)*, Rome, 2004, vol. 6, pp. 3668–3672

134. Y. Wang, E. Vidan, G.W. Bergman, Cardiac motion of coronary arteries: variability in the rest period and implications for coronary MR angiography. Radiology **213**(3), 751–758 (1999)

135. J. Weickert, A. Bruhn, T. Brox, N. Papenberg, *A Survey on Variational Optic Flow Methods for Small Displacements*. Volume 10 of Mathematics in Industry (Springer, Berlin, 2006), pp. 103–136

136. C. Würslin, H. Schmidt, P. Martirosian, C. Brendle, A. Boss, N.F. Schwenzer, L. Stegger, Respiratory motion correction in oncologic PET using T1-weighted MR imaging on a simultaneous whole-body PET/MR system. J. Nucl. Med. **54**(3), 464–471 (2013)

137. D. Yang, H. Li, D.A. Low, J.O. Deasy, I. El Naqa, A fast inverse consistent deformable image registration method based on symmetric optical flow computation. Phys. Med. Biol. **53**(21), 6143 (2008)
138. Y. Yin, E.A. Hoffman, C.L. Lin, Mass preserving nonrigid registration of CT lung images using cubic B-spline. Med. Phys. **36**(9), 4213–4222 (2009)
139. B. Zitova, J. Flusser, Image registration methods: a survey. Image Vis. Comput. **21**(11), 977–1000 (2003)